External Infections of the Eye

External Infections of the Eye

BACTERIAL, VIRAL, AND MYCOTIC

HELENA BIANTOVSKAYA FEDUKOWICZ

Adjunct Associate Professor of Clinical Ophthalmology, New York University School of Medicine; Head of the Eye Microbiology Laboratory, Department of Ophthalmology, Bellevue Hospital, New York

Illustrated by
BEATRICE GROVER

Foreword by
GOODWIN M. BREININ

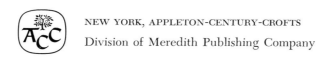

NEW YORK, APPLETON-CENTURY-CROFTS
Division of Meredith Publishing Company

643-1

Library of Congress Card Number: 63-13009

PRINTED IN THE UNITED STATES OF AMERICA

M-30450

This book is dedicated
to students
all over the world

Preface

"One careful observation is worth a thousand alibis."

A modern English treatise on ocular infections including laboratory diagnosis and treatment does not exist. In this day of refined technic and instrumentation, the basic approach to disease and diagnosis has been mislaid. It is my intention to provide not only a reference book on ophthalmic bacteriology, virology, mycology, and cytology but also a practical guide to the study of external ocular diseases.

This book deals primarily with the infectious diseases of the external ocular structures. The more common disease entities are stressed. An approach to understanding the entire disease process and not only the fait accompli (i.e., the end stage of a disease) is attempted. Not only are the biologic characteristics of the offending organisms discussed but also the host characteristics and responses. Each chapter begins with a description of basic general principles. Specific clinical and laboratory findings are then described and correlated. Predisposing factors including age, nutrition, climate, and hygiene are mentioned, for they are important in planning treatment.

Diagnostic methods have been simplified so that they may be used even by the busy practitioner. The therapeutic measures mentioned have been chosen because I have found them to be effective.

References are given at the end of each chapter. Some have historical value. Most others are of recent origin and were gathered primarily from the English language literature.

The practicality of this book is enhanced by numerous illustrations. These with few exceptions are original. Some photographs have been retouched, and some of the paintings have details exaggerated for purposes of emphasis.

The material for the book was developed in the Department of Ophthalmology of the New York University School of Medicine. Thousands of cases of external disease, including those from other clinics and private practice in New York City, have been studied in the laboratory by smear, scraping, and culture, as well as sensitivity and biochemical tests. Records of all these cases were consulted and used in the preparation of this book. The ophthalmic terminology of Duke-Elder is mainly used. I hope that this book will stimulate both students and practicing ophthalmologists to apply basic knowledge and simple laboratory methods to improve diagnosis and treatment of eye infections.

It is impossible to give full acknowledgment for all the help I have received while working on this text. I feel strongly that this book is a collective effort: that of colleagues, students, laboratory workers, librarians, secretaries, and especially of Beatrice Grover, who illustrated the book, and Katherine Sanborn West, who worked closely with me in editing the manuscript. Had either of them faltered during the years of our working together, I could not have finished this book.

I also wish to express deep gratitude to the late Mrs. Antoinette Peterson, who gave indispensable aid in establishing me in my new country.

My profound thanks to:

Dr. Goodwin M. Breinin, Head of the Department of Ophthalmology, for approving the project, reading the manuscript, and for creating the conditions in which our work could be done.

Dr. A. Gerard DeVoe for encouraging and goading me into undertaking the writing.

Dr. Phillips Thygeson for his critical evaluation which led to many helpful changes and additions to the manuscript.

Dr. Alson E. Braley for making this book possible by giving me my first medical appointment in this country.

Dr. George N. Wise for being my good friend and severest critic and spurring me on to make this book better than I knew how.

Dr. Paul Henkind for giving his precious time to help me achieve whatever special qualities this text may have.

Dr. Benjamin Mandel for his valuable criticism of the section on viral infections.

Miss Beatrice Toharsky for her constant availability for consultation, and for her criticism of individual sections on bacterial infections.

Mr. William C. Porth for his immediate understanding and assistance.

Mrs. Joyce Rolls for being a constant source of help in times of stress.

The publisher and editorial staff for exceptional interest and encouragement.

Mr. Walter Lentschner, a photographer of great experience and skill, for producing all the photographs.

The Albert and Mary Lasker Foundation, Allen Grover, and an anonymous donor for their understanding of the educational need for the book and for their generosity in providing funds for the color plates.

HELENA BIANTOVSKAYA FEDUKOWICZ

Contents

Illustrations

Foreword

Dr. Fedukowicz has presented the practitioner, resident, and student of ophthalmology with an integrated textbook of external diseases and micro-biology of the eye. I can think of few areas in ophthalmology where the need has been as pressing. The author brings to this study the experiences of thirteen years as Director of the Laboratory of Ophthalmic Bacteriology at New York University School of Medicine and Bellevue Hospital. Her many years as a practicing ophthalmologist in Europe are reflected in a synthesis of the viewpoints of ophthalmologist and laboratory investigator. Further-more, a long experience in teaching medical students and residents has enabled the author to present the essentials of this subject in a clear and graphic text.

The unified color plates of clinical, bacteriologic, and cytologic data, embellished by Mrs. Grover's artistry, should prove exceedingly useful to all workers in ophthalmology.

GOODWIN M. BREININ

External Infections of the Eye

1

Bacterial External Infections
of the Eye

A FEW GENERAL CONSIDERATIONS

Almost any pathogenic bacteria can cause ocular infection. Certain bacteria, such as the Morax-Axenfeld diplobacillus (*Moraxella lacunata*), *Corynebacterium xerosis*, and the Koch-Weeks bacillus (*Haemophilus aegyptius*), are strictly ophthalmic.

The general principle that infection is determined chiefly by the virulence of the microorganisms and by host resistance applies to the eye. Nevertheless, ocular infections have certain characteristics which result from the unique anatomic structure, physiology, and biochemistry of the eye. Bacteria themselves may undergo some changes in the specific environment of the involved tissue.

Certain bacteria have a special affinity for specific ocular structures; for instance, the gonococcus involves the conjunctiva, with resulting conjunctivitis, but the lacrimal apparatus is never involved; the Koch-Weeks bacillus causes conjunctivitis, but not primary keratitis; *C. xerosis* can grow only on dead epithelium.

External bacterial infections of the eye are usually localized but may frequently spread to adjacent tissue, from the conjunctiva to the cornea, or into the inner eye, or to the orbit, or even to the brain. This is particularly true of streptococcal infections. Some external ocular infections can even be the focus from which metastatic involvement of the body occurs (i.e., from the meningococcus or gonococcus).

Conjunctivitis. Numerous factors protect the conjunctiva from bacterial infection. Among them are: 1, a flushing mechanism provided by tears; 2, the bactericidal action of lysozyme, which is found in tears; 3, phagocytosis, in which the epithelial cells also take part; and 4, the mechanical barrier of an intact mucous membrane. Other factors such as immunity may play a role.

The conjunctiva, being exposed, is the part of the eye most frequently infected. It is sterile at birth but shortly thereafter becomes invaded with various saprophytic bacteria. *C. xerosis* and *Staphylococcus albus* (pages 12 and 28) are regarded as its almost constant inhabitants. Other strains of *Staphylococcus,* the Morax-Axenfeld diplobacillus, the pneumococcus, the Koch-Weeks bacillus, and even streptococci, meningococci, and other organisms may also be found in the so-called normal flora but may be considered potentially pathogenic. All of them, with the exception of *C. xerosis,* may become pathogenic at one time or another. The conjunctiva may harbor many bacteria and thus be a source of infection for other parts of the body or for other individuals. Meningococci are particularly dangerous as they can lead to meningitis of the host or even to meningitis epidemics.

The majority of conjunctival infections are bacterial or viral; fungal infections are rare. The prevalence of specific types of bacteria varies in different regions. Pneumococci and *H. aegyptius* (Koch-Weeks bacillus) are predominantly found in acute conjunctivitis, and staphylococci are found in chronic conjunctivitis.

The inflammatory tissue response to infection is principally of two types: 1, exudative (discharge) and 2, proliferative (follicles or papillary hypertrophy).

The exudate whether predominantly purulent, fibrinous, or hemorrhagic (all types are usually mixed with mucus) is characteristic, though not exclusively so, of a particular bacterial species. The purulent exudate is typically caused by pyogenic bacteria, such as staphylococci and neisseria, and some viruses. The fibrinous exudate, clinically manifested as pseudomembranous or membranous conjunctivitis, is chiefly due to *C. diphtheriae* or hemolytic streptococci. However, membranes can be found in any severe acute conjunctivitis. Hemorrhagic exudation or petechiae possibly indicate hypersensitive reaction to infection. The acute conjunctivitis with exudation is called catarrhalis and is usually a self-limited process of about two weeks duration. Staphylococcal conjunctivitis has a tendency to become chronic.

Since bacterial conjunctivitis is typically an exudative process, the discharge is its most characteristic feature and is the source for transmission of infection.

Secondary corneal involvement may occur in any conjunctivitis. The keratitis is typically marginal and is believed to be due to bacterial allergy or toxin, not to the bacteria themselves. This keratitis is usually not serious and resolves with healing of the conjunctiva. Marginal keratitis is mainly associated with staphylococcal infection.

The epithelial type of keratitis is almost always present in any acute bacterial conjunctivitis. The corneal epithelium is a continuation of the conjunctival epithelium; therefore its involvement may be considered as a part of the conjunctivitis. It must be differentiated from several superficial punctate keratitides of obscure etiology.

The type of exudate, corneal complication, and severity of infection are influenced to a great extent by hygiene, nutrition, and other factors. In certain areas, bacterial conjunctivitis is found to be chiefly purulent with abundant discharge, and it is often associated with secondary keratitis which may be severe.

Children having lymphadenopathy readily develop follicles in any bacterial conjunctivitis. Older individuals respond chiefly by papillary hypertrophy, particularly in long-standing infections. Either reaction may be considered a defense mechanism, differing according to age group.

Blepharitis.   Lid margins are the most common site of staphylococcal infection. Aside from infection, the following factors are of importance in the development of blepharitis: the lid margin acts as an extremity, and circulatory disturbances such as stasis often occur; blond or anemic persons whose skin is sensitive, or individuals with highly vascularized skin, can easily develop red-rimmed eyes. This, while it may predispose to blepharitis, is not in itself a diseased condition. Various irritants both endogenous and exogenous may cause hyperemia. If the irritation persists, stasis occurs, metabolic products collect, and autosensitization may result. The road to inflammation has been laid down. In this favorably disposed condition, bacteria grow readily.

Another factor of importance in the development of blepharitis is that the lashes act as receptacles for dust and bacteria. We thus may say that bacteria are not the only culprits; they must have a favorable environment. Of all the organisms, staphylococci are the prime offenders. *Staphylococcus aureus* is considered pathogenic, while the *albus* variety may or may not be pathogenic.

Blepharitis is characterized by chronicity and may even last a lifetime. The lid margins become rounded and thickened (tylosis ciliaris). The lashes fall out because of hair follicle destruction (madarosis), or the lid margins may become deformed, especially in older persons, resulting in trichiasis or ectropion.

Staphylococcal blepharitis is usually associated with an acute or chronic meibomitis. The organisms are harbored in the glands which act as reservoirs for prolonged infection or sensitization.

Since the condition occurs in poor hygienic surroundings and in cases where resistance is low, the main objectives of treatment must be directed toward improvement of general health and cleanliness of the eye. Removal of scales and crusts before further treatment is mandatory. The patient should wash his face at least twice a day with hot water and soap.

Seborrheic blepharitis is even more troublesome and more frequent than is staphylococcal blepharitis. Hypersecretion of the sebaceous glands in seborrhea is usually generalized; in older persons, it may be a local process, either hypersecretion or atonic retention of the meibomian glands. The normal cholesterol fats change to cholesterol esters; the latter support growth, particularly of *Pityrosporum ovale* and staphylococci. These aggravate the seborrheic blepharitis, which then may become ulcerative. Without this, seborrheic blepharitis is a mild process characterized by greasy scales. The foamy secretion along the lid margin is a sign of hypersecretion of the meibomian glands.

The expression of the secretion, simultaneously with massage, has primary importance in treatment. The patient, properly instructed, can do it himself.

Keratitis. The cornea is a unique anatomic structure. It consists of a hard homogeneous avascular tissue which is incapable of regeneration (except the epithelial and endothelial cells and Descemet's membrane). The predominant feature of corneal infection is a necrosis, often with resulting ulcer formation. Damage, unless extremely mild, leaves its permanent mark on the cornea.

There are two main types of keratitis in which bacteria have to be considered: marginal and central hypopyon. Marginal keratitis, while common in bacterial conjunctivitis, is rarely caused by the bacteria themselves but is rather a secondary toxic or hypersensitivity response.

Central infectious keratitis generally follows corneal trauma and is due to direct invasion by bacteria. The process is usually severe, and destruction of the eye may be the consequence. The severity of the process depends upon two factors: 1, virulence of the invading organism; 2, position of the infection in the center of the cornea which is most exposed, most sensitive, thinnest, and above all, most poorly nourished and poorly supplied by antibodies. This keratitis is usually purulent; an infiltrate of yellowish color is characteristically noted. It is accompanied by a sterile hypopyon which indicates that toxin is infiltrating into the anterior chamber and causing an iritis. There is a purulent conjunctivitis which is secondary to the keratitis.

The most common organism found in central hypopyon keratitis is the pneumococcus. The gram-negative bacilli, particularly of the enteric group, are also increasingly recognized as a cause of this keratitis. At Bellevue Hospital we have noted a very high incidence of moraxella keratitis. Clinically, pneumococcal keratitis is serpiginous, spreading along the surface. The active, progressive edge of the ulcer is usually undermined. The material for laboratory investigation must be taken from this pocket where the bacteria have accumulated. Keratitis due to *Moraxella lacunata* or to other gram-negative bacilli, such as the enteric group (particularly *Pseudomonas aeruginosa*), is abscesslike, spreading deeply. When caused by *Ps. aeruginosa* (*B. pyocyaneus*) the process may become fulminating, resulting in perforation or even panophthalmitis.

The prognosis for central bacterial keratitis is always guarded, particularly in that due to gram-negative bacilli, most of which are resistant to antibiotics.

Dacryocystitis. The basis for this infection is a blockage of the duct system. The flushing mechanism is disturbed, and tear fluid collects in the lacrimal sac. The tears, which have served to clear the eye, wash the bacteria into the sac where they may readily multiply. Among the micro-organisms, often mixed, that may be found are staphylococci, viridans streptococci, *Neisseria catarrhalis*, the Koch-Weeks bacillus, *Ps. aeruginosa*, and others. The pneumococcus is the most common inhabitant. This condition must be considered a very dangerous reservoir of infection.

Two main types of dacryocystitis exist: chronic and acute. A number of different types of bacteria are usually found in the chronic type. They do not cause a visible inflammatory process and hence the condition may be overlooked. The microorganisms become very virulent in injured tissue, resulting in acute dacryocystitis or severe hypopyon keratitis.

If the lacrimal tissue is injured, an acute dacryocystitis may ensue. Probing the lacrimal apparatus must be carefully done to avoid injury to its components. If the infection does not clear under medical management, surgical procedures are necessary. If hypopyon keratitis occurs, immediate removal of the lacrimal sac may be indicated.

2

Bacteria

MORPHOLOGIC CHARACTERISTICS OF BACTERIA

EXTERNAL STRUCTURE

Cell Wall. This is the rigid outer layer of the bacterium. Chemically it consists of proteins, carbohydrates, and lipids.

Cytoplasmic Membrane. This is the concentrated peripheral part of the cytoplasm, adjusting to the inner surface of the cell wall.

Being semipermeable membranes, the cell wall and the cytoplasmic membrane both serve as osmotic barriers between the external and internal environments of the bacterial cells. These structures have many other characteristics, such as antigenic properties and electric charge (tendency of bacteria to migrate in an electric field).

Capsule. This superficial slime layer surrounds the bacterial cell wall (it appears as a clear zone, especially in stained preparation). It is suggested that, depending upon environment, practically all bacteria can develop capsules. The degree of encapsulation differs; some have a well-developed capsule, others an almost invisible one. However, in certain bacteria, capsules are constantly present. This is probably a matter of heredity. Some bacteria develop a capsule only in tissue (i.e., *Clostridium perfringens*), some in both tissue and culture (the pneumococcus and *Klebsiella pneumoniae*).

Chemically, the capsular material is not a permanent structure. In many species, the capsule consists of polysaccharides which stimulate the formation of antibodies in tissues. In certain groups of pneumococci, *Klebsiella pneumoniae* and *Haemophilus influenzae,* the capsular carbohydrates also determine the specificity of the serologic groups. Medical bacteriologists used to correlate the presence of a capsule with virulence (the capsule serves as a means of protection for the pathogens, mainly against phagocytosis).

Flagella. These are the organs of motion. Some bacteria are able to move throughout their life; others are motile only during certain periods of cell development. Flagella are cytoplasmic processes extending through the pores in the cell wall and chemically composed of proteins. They are very thin, usually longer than the body, and are arranged in various patterns on the bacterial cell, one or more in number.

A number of bacteria (most bacilli, spirilla, and some coccal forms, particularly saprophytic) have flagella. Not all motile bacteria move by means of flagella—spirochetes seem to swim like snakes. There is no connection between flagellar motility and tissue invasion nor with pathogenicity in general.

The active motion also can be due to impulses originating in the bacteria themselves.

INTERNAL STRUCTURE

Nucleus.   The presence of a nucleus in bacteria was established only recently. Opinions have ranged from complete denial that a bacterial nucleus exists to the assumption that the entire bacterial cell is a nucleus. The process of transmission of hereditary factors in bacteria confirms the existence of nuclear material. Demonstration of a bacterial nucleus is difficult because most bacteria contain large amounts of ribonucleic acid (RNA) which masks the real nucleic material—desoxyribonucleic acid (DNA)— because RNA has the same high sensitivity to basic dyes as DNA. Demonstration of nucleic material is possible after the removal of RNA by the enzyme ribonuclease. Then the Feulgen reaction which is specific for DNA is often positive in bacterial structures. These structures do not represent a typical nucleus of higher organisms; they do not have typical chromosomes and they multiply not by mitosis but by simple division of the nucleus into two daughter fragments. However, on the basis of recent data, the possible presence of chromosomes is assumed.

Cytoplasmic Elements.   Bacterial cytoplasm is a structureless colloidal mixture of enzymes and metabolites with a variety of granules.

Volutin Granules.   These are also known as metachromatic granules, Babes-Ernst granules, and ribonucleic acid granules. Common in most bacteria, they occur in the form of refractile granules having the same high affinity to basic dyes as does chromatin material. Volutin granules are not a permanent structure and may disappear completely after starvation of bacteria; on this basis they are regarded as food storage for bacteria. The presence of volutin granules is significant for diagnosis and for differentiation of bacterial species, particularly the *Corynebacterium* species.

Carbohydrates.   Reserve polysaccharide-glycogen and starch granules are found in many bacterial species. They may be regarded as food storage. The granules are identified by staining with iodine.

Fats and Lipids.   Their globules are a common finding in bacteria, being particularly abundant in acid-fast bacilli. The very refractile and intensely stained fat globules resemble chromatin material or endospores.

Spores. Sporulation of bacteria generally occurs in an unfavorable environment (e.g., a dry one). As soon as spores again find good conditions they germinate into fresh vegetative cells. Spores are seen in unstained films as highly refractive spherical bodies surrounded by light zones; they may be seen in stained films only when spore membranes are permeable. Most yeasts, molds, and many bacilli produce spores, while most cocci do not produce them. Usually only a single spore develops, occasionally two. In some bacteria (*Clostridia*) the spores cause a bulge. Filamentous bacteria (e.g., *Nocardia*) may produce spores termed conidia, which very closely resemble the spores of molds.

Chemically, spores are rich in lipids and apparently contain a large amount of chromatinlike nuclear material.

Size. Next to viruses and rickettsiae, bacteria are the smallest living organisms, and their small size is their most characteristic property. However, there is great variation in size (range: 0.1 to 50 microns); the majority of bacteria studied in the laboratory are between 0.5 and 2 microns. Size is influenced by hereditary characteristics and environmental factors.

Size has a great effect on the behavior of bacteria; volume and surface area are important factors in the process of diffusion and elimination of waste products. The smaller the bacteria, the less complex is their structure; they are apt to be deficient in enzymes and hence more dependent upon the host cells. The antigenic properties of smaller bacteria have a more definite action. The larger species of a genus have a lower temperature growth range than the small ones. A bacterial population that has passed beyond the stage of its maximum growth rate consists of smaller bacteria than a young culture; only corynebacteria are smaller in young culture.

Size is the main determining factor in the segmentation of bacteria. As the bulk of a bacterium is increased, the surface becomes proportionately smaller, and then arises the necessity for segmentation or subdivision of the organism.

Shape. Three main morphologic groups are recognized: coccal or spheroidal (including lancet, flattened, and kidney-shaped), bacillary or cylindrical, and spiral. The variety of shapes may be very marked; bacillary, coccal, and filamentous forms may all be present in the same species, which is then called pleomorphic. Age, environment, species, and even the technic of preparing the specimen are important determinants of shape.

Grouping or Arrangement. When a bacterial cell divides, the two daughter cells may remain attached to one another by their cell membrane, or they may separate immediately. Depending on the plane and number of divisions and the tendency to remain together, various arrangements occur. It is a general rule that the division of bacteria takes place at a right angle to the longest axis of the cell; it is transverse, not longitudinal. In cocci, the division may occur in any plane, since a sphere has no longest axis. As a result, cocci show a greater variety of grouping than do bacilli. Among the cocci the diplo or strepto arrangement is the result of parallel division, tetra is the result of division in two planes, sarcine in three planes, and cluster results from irregular division. Among the bacilli, which are always divided perpendicularly to their long axis, the arrangement occurs typically in diplo-bacillary and streptobacillary forms. The chain arrangement in bacilli has no such inference of pathogenicity as in cocci formation. In some bacteria (*Corynebacterium*) a postfission movement occurs which can bring the cells into parallel or palisade arrangement.

Since the grouping of bacteria may be much influenced by physical and mechanical factors in their environment, arrangement itself is not suffi-ciently significant for diagnosis. Arrangement however, together with typical shape and staining, may be of determinative value.

Reproduction. This can occur during the active vegetative or resting stage. The usual method of multiplication is by simple binary fission, which occurs as a transverse, never longitudinal, segmentation of bacteria. There are other ways of multiplication than fission: sporulation, budding, and sexual reproduction. Spores are reproductive bodies. The sexual type of reproduction is relatively primitive, due to the primitive structure of the nucleus.

HOST-PARASITE RELATIONSHIP

A great variety of factors characterizes the ability of a microorganism to establish disease in a given host. It is impossible to mention all of them, even briefly.

The most important principle is that the infectious agent must be able to penetrate the protective cellular and humoral barriers of the host and to find a favorable environment for multiplication. To destroy the protective barrier, the infectious agent must be virulent. Virulence is determined by a great number of complex factors. Most important among these are invasive-ness and toxigenicity.

Invasiveness. Many diseases develop not because of toxin but pri-marily because of invasiveness—the ability of microorganisms to enter the body and to spread throughout the tissues (e.g., anthrax and plague bacilli invade tissue rapidly and multiply extensively in most tissues).

ENZYMES play a leading role in the process of invasiveness. Knowledge of their action is incomplete. A brief description of some of them will be given:

Hyaluronidase is a spreading factor which hydrolyzes hyaluronic acid, a cementing substance of tissue. It also hydrolyzes a capsular component of certain bacteria.

Streptokinase is a proteolytic enzyme produced by certain hemolytic streptococci. It dissolves human fibrin clots, which action is indirect. It is believed that streptokinase activates plasminogen, which is a precursor of plasmin, a proteolytic ferment in plasma.

Streptodornase is a streptococcal desoxyribonuclease enzyme which lowers the viscosity of DNA. The viscosity of purulent exudate depends largely upon the desoxyribonuclease proteins. A mixture of streptodornase and streptokinase is used to liquefy exudates and to break down the fibrin barrier, especially in narrow spaces.

Coagulase coagulates plasma to form a wall around staphylococcal lesions. It also protects staphylococci from phagocytosis by a deposit of fibrin on the surface of bacteria.

A number of toxic and nontoxic substances are elaborated by pathogenic bacteria during their growth. These are hemolysin, fibrinolysin, leukocidin, erythrogenic toxin, and others.

Toxigenicity. This is due to toxins, which are subdivided into exotoxins and endotoxins.

Exotoxins are liberated into surrounding tissues by many gram-positive (rarely gram-negative) bacteria without destroying themselves. Exotoxins have a specific effect on certain cells of the host (e.g., tetanus toxin affects motor nerve cells). Exotoxins stimulate the production of antibodies (in amounts proportional to the toxin) and are specifically neutralized by them. They can also be converted into toxoids (antigenic but nonpoisonous) by heat, formalin, and prolonged storage.

Endotoxins are intimately associated with most gram-negative bacteria. They can be liberated into the surrounding medium only by autolysis of bacteria (not by simple filtration). Chemically, endotoxins are lipid-polysaccharide-polypeptides which are identical to the O antigen, type-specific of enteric bacilli (found in the bodies of bacteria and equally efficient in the production of antibodies as a whole bacterium). Endotoxins are seldom antigenic, which makes it difficult to prepare anti-endotoxin sera. They do not cause characteristic diseases in experimental animals. Endotoxins are relatively heat-stable. Endotoxins of most gram-negative bacilli are similar, as are their pharmacologic and pathologic effects. Therefore, the existence of a common toxic component is assumed. Antibiotics have no effect on most of the gram-negative bacilli.

In the ability of a parasite to produce infection, a variety of other factors play important roles. The route of introduction of the infectious agent modifies the virulence (very toxic tetanus is harmless when swallowed; many bacteria nonpathogenic in intact tissue become very virulent in injured tissue). The site of the primary lesion and the direction of initial spread of infection (particularly by the direction of lymphatic flow) are largely determined by the portal of entry. However, the biochemical environment of the host tissue (resistance and immunity) ultimately determines the production of infection.

Resistance and Immunity. Resistance is determined by humoral and cellular defense barriers of the host, in which two groups of factors must be considered: nonspecific and specific.

Nonspecific factors include defense barriers at the portal of entry (skin and mucous membranes with their secretory glands), phagocytosis, inflammatory response, and biochemical tissue constituents.

Specific factors include various forms of immunity:

1. Natural immunity—racial, individual, and species immunity.
2. Acquired immunity, which is subdivided into active and passive:

Active immunity, a state wherein the host itself actively produces antibodies following introduction of live or killed microorganisms, antigens, toxins, or toxoids. This type of immunity lasts for years.

Passive immunity, acquired passively by introduction of antibodies from another host. As a result, this immunity is only temporary.

Lack of resistance to infection is termed susceptibility.

In many infections, the allergic state plays an important or dominant role. Allergy can be divided roughly into immediate and delayed types. However, these are not always sharply distinguishable.

Delayed reaction develops within no less than 12 to 48 hours and progresses for two to three days or longer. It is characterized by absence of circulating antibodies in the serum. A cellular mechanism is suggested. It is known to be specific and is capable of specific desensitization. It cannot be transferred by serum, but recent data show possible transfer by cells, particularly the white cells.

The tuberculin reaction is a classical type of delayed allergy. A tuberculinlike sensitivity may be induced by almost any type of protein. Delayed allergy occurs more frequently in certain chronic infections—bacterial, viral, or fungal. According to Smith and Conant (page 212):

Spontaneous sensitization of this type occurs regularly in tuberculosis, typhoid fever, glanders, brucellosis, pneumococcal pneumonia, chancroid, echinococcus infection, streptococcal infections, lymphogranuloma venereum, coccidioidomycosis, histoplasmosis, mumps, and vaccinia virus.

Bacterial infection may be complicated by either immediate or delayed sensitivity.

The sensitivity to infection is usually termed bacterial allergy.

The delayed type is recognized in many conditions other than infections and is usually manifested as a dermatitis, such as contact dermatitis. The classical example of this is dermatitis due to contact with poison ivy. Certain drugs and many chemicals used in manufacturing processes produce contact dermatitis. In many of these cases, antigens are incomplete or haptene, commonly polysaccharide in naturally occurring antigens or low molecular weight substances in artificial antigens. They do not stimulate antibody production but, being combined with host proteins, may become complete antigens.

An immediate hypersensitivity reaction is a response to the artificial introduction (injection) of allergens. It may develop within two or three minutes or may take several hours. The reaction is usually acute and systemic. The antigen-antibody reaction takes place in the serum and can be transmitted. Anaphylaxis is the classical type of immediate reaction which is systemic. Arthus's phenomenon is an example of local immediate reaction.

Predisposing factors—hunger, thirst, heat, cold, fatigue, hygiene, and resistance of the host—must be considered. For a more detailed study of such a complex subject as immunity and allergy, readers are referred to special texts.

REFERENCES

1. Axenfeld, T. A.   The Bacteriology of the Eye, London, Baillière, Tindall and Cox, 1908.
2. Breed, R. S., Murray, E. G. D., and Smith, N. R.   Bergey's Manual of Determinative Bacteriology, 7th ed., Baltimore, Williams & Wilkins Co., 1957.
3. Cason, L., and Winkler, C. H., Jr.   Bacteriology of the eye. I. Normal flora, Arch. Ophth., 51:196, 1954; Winkler, C. H., Jr., and Cason, L. II. Role of gram-negative bacilli in infections following cataract extraction, Arch. Ophth., 51:200, 1954.
4. Dubos, R. J.   Bacterial and Mycotic Infections of Man, 3rd ed., Philadelphia, J. B. Lippincott Co., 1958.
5. Duke-Elder, W. S.   Text-book of Ophthalmology, St. Louis, C. V. Mosby Co., 1946, vol. 2.
6. Norn, M. S.   A quantitative method for studying the cytology of the conjunctiva, Acta ophth., 36:502, 1958.
7. Rich, A. R.   Experimental pathological studies on the nature and role of bacterial allergy, Acta paediat., 16:1, 1933.
8. Sery, T. W.   Recent advances in ocular microbiology, Surv. Ophth., 4:425, 1959.
9. Smith, D. T., and Conant, N. F.   Zinsser Microbiology, 12th ed., New York, Appleton-Century-Crofts, Inc., 1960.
10. Soudakoff, P. S.   Bacteriologic examination of the conjunctiva, Am. J. Ophth., 38:374, 1954.
11. Theodore, F. H., and Schlossman, A.   Ocular Allergy, Baltimore, Williams & Wilkins Co., 1958.
12. Thomas, C. I.   The Cornea, Springfield, Ill., Charles C Thomas Publisher, 1955.
13. Thygeson, P.   The cytology of conjunctival exudates, Am. J. Ophth., 29:1499, 1946.
14. ———   Marginal corneal infiltrates and ulcers, Arch. Ophth., 39:432, 1948.
15. Woods, A. C.   The diagnosis and treatment of ocular allergy, Am. J. Ophth., 32:1457, 1949.
16. Wright, R. E.   Superficial punctate keratitis, Brit. J. Ophth., 14:257, 1930.

GRAM-POSITIVE GROUP

PYOGENIC COCCI

The Staphylococci

Staphylococcus is a genus of the family *Micrococcaceae*. Staphylococci are actual or potential pathogens, being constant inhabitants of the skin and most mucous membranes, including the conjunctiva. They produce a variety of infections, ranging from a mild carbuncle to fatal septicemia. Primarily a causative agent of pyogenic infections, they also have the ability to necrotize tissue. They are usually characterized by abscess formation.

Any structure of the body can be invaded by staphylococci. In ocular infections, staphylococci occupy first place among all organisms.

The staphylococcal infections are usually sporadic, not epidemic. Their chronicity presents a difficult problem for treatment. The dramatic effect of penicillin when first introduced has now created a serious problem. Staphylococcal strains resistant to penicillin isolated from hospital patients and personnel have increased over 75 per cent in less than 15 years (Smith and Conant). As a result, some infections such as staphylococcal enteritis have become highly fatal.

Morphology. Staphylococci are typically gram-positive, extracellular, spherical, arranged in clusters, and do not possess a capsule (Plate I, 5B). However, they vary in size, shape, and staining ability. In smear of the secretion, they can be intracellular, flattened on one side, and arranged singly, in pairs, or in short chains (Plate I, 5A). There is also individual variation in resistance to decoloration by the gram method. As a result, gram-negative strains occur. Besides, some staphylococci are naturally gram-negative. All these variations often make diagnosis in direct smear impossible. This is feasible only in the case of typical morphologic characteristics, such as spherical shape, definite gram-positive stain, and cluster arrangement. Culture is always necessary to confirm diagnosis and to test virulence and sensitivity.

Culture. Staphylococci grow readily on all ordinary bacteriologic media. Colonies are easily identified on solid media. They are typically opaque, round, discrete (not mucoid), smooth, raised, glistening, and from 1 to 2 mm in diameter. In smear from the culture, the morphology varies depending on whether the medium is solid or fluid, or the culture young or old.

The colonies show active pigment production. In the presence of oxygen, pigment production is enhanced, especially on agar containing carbohydrates. Also to be noted is that an incubation temperature of 22° C is more conducive to pigment production than the usual incubation temperature of 37° C.

Three types of staphylococci were originally distinguished by their differences in pigmentation: 1, *Staphylococcus aureus*, yellowish golden; 2, *Staphylococcus albus*, white; and 3, *Staphylococcus citreus*, lemon-yellow (Plate I, 6). However, all of these are grayish white in young culture.

It was once considered that *Staphylococcus aureus* was the only pathogenic strain. Recent studies show that S. *albus* can be pathogenic. Therefore confusion of nomenclature has arisen.

Staphylococcus is classified as Genus II of the family *Micrococcaceae* in the seventh edition of *Bergey's Manual of Determinative Bacteriology*, 1957. The type species is *Staphylococcus aureus* Rosenbach. Bergey's considers *Staphylococcus albus* as a white variety of *Staphylococcus aureus* and states that the name *Staphylococcus albus* should never be used for any white staphylococci. Unfortunately, this statement is made without discussion of pathogenicity of this variety. In our laboratory, the coagulase test was constantly positive in the *aureus* strain and only occasionally positive in the *albus* strain. Also, *aureus* is usually isolated from diseases, but *albus* is frequently found in the normal flora. The most recent editions of both Dubos and Smith and Conant state that *Staphylococcus aureus* is more pathogenic than *albus*. Tests for pathogenicity of staphylococci include: fermentation of mannitol, liquefaction of gelatin, and production of coagulase. The coagulase test is more conclusive for pathogenicity.

On blood agar, staphylococci may produce hemolysis which is apparently not concerned directly with pathogenicity, as is the case with streptococcal hemolysis.

The virulence of pathogenic strains is generally, but not always, diminished by prolonged cultivation. Even after years of subculture in the laboratory the virulence may remain intact. Moreover animal passage may enhance the virulence of the pathogenic strains but has not induced virulence in saprophytic strains.

COAGULASE TEST. The technic can be simplified as follows: citrated plasma is mixed on a microscope slide with a suspension of staphylococci. With pathogenic strains the suspension becomes coagulated (Plate II, 3).

Staphylococci are hardy microorganisms in spite of the fact that they are not sporeformers. Staphylococci can be dried and still reproduce.

TOXINS AND ENZYMES. Most of the pathogenic staphylococci produce various toxins. They are: lethal toxins causing death of animals when injected intravenously; leukocidin, destroying leukocytes (its role in pathogenicity is uncertain); enterotoxin, causing acute gastroenteritis (food poisoning); and others.

Coagulase, an enzyme produced by staphylococci, coagulates fibrin. This forms a wall around the individual staphylococci and around the lesions. Hence phagocytosis is prevented and a delimited abscess usually develops.

There are many other extracellular substances, among them hyaluronidase (spreading factor), proteinase, and lipase.

Toxoid may be readily prepared from staphylococcal exotoxins. The toxoid stimulates antibody formation and is used in treatment.

Pathology. In general, staphylococci produce localized abscesses. It must be remembered, however, that the pathology also depends upon the route of introduction and the tissue involved. For example, if staphylococci are introduced upon the skin or mucous membrane, the resultant inflammation is usually chronic or mildly acute. On the other hand, if staphylococci are introduced beneath skin or mucous membranes, an acute process and abscess formation evolve. The main reason is probably that the skin and mucous membranes are constantly inhabited by staphylococci and thereby develop a resistance to the organisms.

The discharge is usually purulent, even in mild infections of the mucous membranes. It may be abundant without much tissue involvement. The bacteria proliferate upon the surface without invading it. The organism is not found in living epithelium and is seldom phagocytized.

In the consideration of chronic recurrent staphylococcal infections, host resistance or hypersensitivity would seem even more important than bacterial virulence.

Findings in the Eye. Staphylococci are the most common, as well as the most thoroughly studied, cause of ocular infections. Not long ago, staphylococci were regarded simply as harmless conjunctival saprophytes. It is thus significant that experiments have established that ophthalmic staphylococci produce powerful toxins.[1] The development of tests for pathogenicity is also of major importance.[29] With the advent of antibiotics we can now successfully treat *acute* staphylococcal infections, especially cellulitis, which were previously dangerous. However, treatment of *chronic* staphylococcal infections and prevention of their recurrence are still a serious problem in ophthalmology. The importance of allergic reactions to staphylococcal infections is now frequently discussed; all staphylococci may be antigenic. Unfortunately, allergy cannot be satisfactorily proven until the various types of sensitization are more fully understood (Theodore and Schlossman).[30]

Two factors which are deemed important though not sufficiently stressed in the literature are: resistance of the body or local tissue, which in any chronic process is of primary importance, and local ocular hygiene. In low resistance, it is known that susceptibility is higher to any kind of stimulating or irritating factors, and the term susceptibility would appear preferable to hypersensitivity.

Local hygiene of the eye can be remarkably effective without any other treatment. This includes removal of scales and crusts from lid margins. Simply washing the face with hot water and mild soap, morning and night, can markedly improve the condition. Unfortunately, antibiotic ointment is often applied on top of heavy crusts.

Of all staphylococcal ocular diseases, blepharitis is the most common.

BLEPHARITIS.   Two clinical forms are seen: ulcerative (Plate I, 1), and squamous. Staphylococci play a primary role in the ulcerative form and a secondary role in the squamous type, which is usually seborrheic, and here the staphylococcus acts as a secondary invader. Either type may recur and persist for years. The condition is usually associated with conjunctivitis and purulent inflammation of the hair follicles as well as of the adjacent meibomian glands (hordeolum externum and internum). Bacteria accumulated under the crusts of the ulcer or inside the meibomian glands [28] result in a process of long duration and, often, hypersensitivity of tissue. Tylosis ciliaris (thickening of the lid margins) and madarosis (loss of cilia) caused by destruction of the hair follicles are unpleasant complications of the process (Plate II, 1).

CONJUNCTIVITIS.   In adults, conjunctivitis is usually chronic and secondary to blepharitis. Involvement of the tarsal portion is pathognomonic for blepharitis, which is sometimes unnoticed, especially when mild.

Acute conjunctivitis, seen usually in children, is less frequent than the chronic and may develop independently of the blepharitis (Plate I, 4). This has a rather typical appearance: 1, the lower palpebral conjunctiva is predominantly infected; 2, the discharge may be scanty or heavy; however, the underlying tissue is little involved; 3, the condition is initially acute and if not properly treated may easily become chronic; and 4, corneal complications are not infrequent.

At this point, we must mention acute staphylococcal conjunctivitis of the newborn (ophthalmia neonatorum), for this differs from the condition as manifested in later life. This condition occasionally reminds one of gonoblennorrhea. Corneal involvement is unknown, and there is no tendency to chronicity. The explanation of these peculiarities probably lies in some anatomic characteristics (absence of lymphatic tissue in the conjunctiva and rudimentary meibomian glands).

Phlyctenules are a frequent reaction to staphylococcal conjunctivitis, particularly in children. The lesions often ulcerate.

Children with lymphatic adenopathy often develop follicles, which may be numerous, predominantly in the lower fornix.

KERATITIS. Surprisingly, primary central staphylococcal hypopyon keratitis rarely results from corneal injury. The keratitis usually develops secondary to staphylococcal conjunctivitis or blepharoconjunctivitis.

The most frequent type is marginal (Plate I, 3), characterized by a small, grayish infiltrate adjacent to but often separated from the limbus by a narrow clear zone. The small, multiple infiltrates may run along the entire limbus. The infiltrated area ulcerates readily. The process may be caused by staphylococcal toxin, and bacteria are usually not found in the scraping from the ulcer. The keratitis is mild and is generally cured together with the conjunctivitis.

Superficial punctate keratitis also may complicate staphylococcal infection. Tiny punctate epithelial erosions, most marked in the lower half of the cornea, can be seen only by staining with fluorescein. The condition is most often observed in acute staphylococcal conjunctivitis, being probably an allergic reaction. This also can be regarded as part of the process in the conjunctiva.

HORDEOLUM. Hordeolum internum is an acute inflammation of the meibomian glands, mainly caused by staphylococci (Plate I, 2). The process is stubbornly resistant to treatment (drugs do not readily penetrate the glands). Hordeolum externum (acute inflammation of the Zeis glands) is also usually a staphylococcal infection. The process is more accessible to treatment. If it is localized at the angulus externus, a tremendous edema may develop, as the lymphatic ways cross here. *Hordeolosum*, the persistent recurrence of several hordeola, may be seen in patients with chronic blepharitis or conjunctivitis or in debilitated persons.

Staphylococci can also cause such dangerous diseases as orbital cellulitis and intraocular postoperative infection.[6]

Staphylococci are the most common secondary invaders in many conditions: dacryocystitis, trachoma, pemphigus, keratomalacia, measles, and some others. Most frequently staphylococcal infections of the eye are associated with skin diseases.

Treatment. Fortunately, resistant strains have not as yet presented a great problem in ophthalmology. However, the sensitivity test is necessary in all chronic and acute cases to insure the proper choice of antibiotics. Such therapy, to be successful, depends upon many additional factors. The medication should be discontinued if there is no response within a few days. Treatment with a particular antibiotic must immediately be stopped if sensitivity develops, and perhaps another used in its place.

While we must be concerned with proper treatment, it should be strongly emphasized that many cases are overtreated, and this may sometimes seriously complicate the picture.

Toxoid therapy should be tried in chronic recurrent infections if other therapy has failed.[16, 32]

Staphylococcal antitoxin is of value only in cases of toxemia.

Regardless of any method of treatment, in blepharitis the lid margins must first be cleaned. The simplest method is to use hot compresses (with hot water or carbonate lotion or saline solution) for 5 to 10 minutes. The softened scales and crusts are then removed. Epilation of the lashes is indicated if there is suppuration of the hair follicles. Following these procedures, a variety of medication may be applied to the lids. Painting the lid margins with silver nitrate (1 per cent or 2 per cent) or with brilliant green * (1 per cent in 70 per cent alcohol) is valuable in blepharitis. Expressing the secretion from the meibomian glands and employing massage are highly recommended, especially in squamous blepharitis.

Attention to the health of the patient (good diet and hygiene—washing the face morning and night with hot water and mild soap) is helpful. Such predisposing factors as any kind of irritation must be considered.

The Streptococci

These are gram-positive cocci, typically arranged in chains. Streptococci cause a variety of severe diseases in man, among them scarlet fever, erysipelas, septicemia, infection of surgical wounds (sometimes fatal), cellulitis, puerperal fever, and epidemic sore throat. The incidence of streptococcal infection increases in the winter.

Streptococci also play an important role in various serious ocular infections, particularly cellulitis.

Allergy to streptococci or their products may be significant in rheumatic

* Apply brilliant green to the dried lid margin with a toothpick applicator, using a minimum amount of the stain.

fever, nephritis, and endocarditis, and in such diseases of the eye as irido-cyclitis.

There are a number of classifications of streptococci, two of which have received marked attention. Brown classified streptococci according to their action on blood agar: the alpha type, known also as *viridans* streptococci, produces a greenish incomplete hemolysis; beta streptococci, known as the *hemolyticus* group, produce complete hemolysis; and the gamma type, known as *Streptococcus nonhemolyticus,* has no hemolytic effect. Of the streptococci to be discussed here, *Streptococcus pyogenes* shows beta he-molysis, *Streptococcus mitis* shows alpha hemolysis, and *Streptococcus sali-varius* is nonhemolytic.

Lancefield divides the hemolytic streptococci into groups based on their antigenic properties. There are distinguished 13 serologic groups, or more, from A to O. The majority pathogenic for man fall into group A.

This serologic typing is more valuable than hemolysis in the study of individual characteristics of streptococci. For practical reasons, however, in medical laboratories identification according to the type of hemolysis is still a routine procedure.

We shall discuss the pathogenic strains as a whole.

Morphology. Streptococci are gram-positive, round or elongated cocci, usually flattened at adjacent sides. The organisms are typically arranged in long chains consisting of eight or more cocci. The long chains are found in smear from exudate or in fluid media. However extremely long chains may appear. On solid media, streptococci occur in pairs, short chains, or groups, closely resembling those of staphylococci (Plate VI, 3). The cocci vary greatly in size and staining. In old culture, club-shaped or gram-negative organisms may occur.

Encapsulation is not a typical characteristic of streptococci. When it does appear, it is more likely to be in members of group A or certain mem-bers of group C. The capsule lasts only for about the first two to two and a half hours of growth and disappears very quickly. There is probably no connection between encapsulation and virulence.

Culture. Streptococci require enriched media; on ordinary media, growth is poor. Blood agar plates are routinely used for primary isolation and determination of the type of hemolysis. The hemolysis is influenced by the blood used. Horse or rabbit blood is best and the medium should be glucose-free. On blood agar, colonies are pinpoint, grayish, and slightly opalescent, resembling small droplets of fluid and surrounded by a zone of hemolysis (incomplete in alpha; complete and sharply defined in beta). The minute colonies and big zone (2 to 4 mm) of hemolysis are important diagnostic characteristics (Plate VI, 2). Nevertheless, the size of the hemolytic zone varies considerably.

Depending upon the phase of dissociation, colonies may vary from the slimy mucoid types to granular or even dry.

Antigenic Structure.   Many antigens have been isolated: group-specific carbohydrates, proteins, and nucleoproteins. Carbohydrates are contained in the cell wall of many streptococci. These are the most important substances for serologic grouping of streptococci. In relation to the antigenic substances, 13 serologic groups (Lancefield A to O) are distinguished.

Pathogenicity.   Pathogenicity is due to a variety of active substances, toxins and enzymes, elaborated by streptococci. Enzymes are the determining factors in pathogenicity, causing a marked invasiveness. They are as follows:

Streptokinase is an enzyme which dissolves human fibrin clots. Its action is indirect, but it is supposed that streptokinase activates plasminogen, which is a precursor of plasmin, a proteolytic ferment in plasma.

Streptodornase (desoxyribonuclease) lowers the viscosity of the exudate which has been caused by desoxyribonucleic acid (DNA). Streptodornase is closely related to streptococcal streptokinase. They have been employed clinically, individually or together, in a variety of conditions requiring enzymatic debridement. However, since both may be toxic, other enzymes, such as dornase, are preferred.

Hyaluronidase (spreading factor) splits hyaluronic acid, the substance cementing together connective tissue. Hyaluronidase is particularly responsible for diffusely spreading streptococcal infections.

Hemolysins, streptolysins, leukocidins, and erythrogenic toxins are also responsible for pathogenicity.

Pathology.   In contrast to staphylococcal infections, streptococcal infections are serous or serosanguineous and usually insuppurative. The infection is generally diffuse and rapidly spreading, due to enzymes. The pyogenic process appears in the form of cellulitis rather than the localized abscess which is typical for staphylococcal infections. Very often the focal infection becomes generalized and septicemic. Focal streptococcal infections, commonly pharyngitis or tonsillitis, may be responsible for a variety of systemic diseases, such as endocarditis, rheumatic fever, and rheumatoid arthritis. The mechanism is not clear: the possibility of hypersensitivity to bacterial toxins, rather than bacterial infections, has to be considered.

Findings in the Eye.   Cellulitis of the lid is most commonly caused by *Streptococcus pyogenes.* The eyebrow line is a usual site of infection. The process is generally associated with injury and may rarely follow metastasis of bacteria from distant parts of the body. It is characterized initially by localized infiltration and severe swelling. The process progresses rapidly, and massive necrosis may follow (Plate VI, 4). The infection may spread into the orbit or even into the brain or down the face.

Orbital cellulitis due to *Streptococcus pyogenes,* prevalent in children, results chiefly from sinusitis or focal infections of the teeth or from pharyngitis. Panophthalmitis may ensue. The cellulitis may also be complicated by cavernous sinus thrombosis, which is always serious and can even be fatal.

Streptococcal panophthalmitis, postoperative or following injury, may occur (Plate VI, 5).

Lacrimal sac abscess due to streptococci, while uncommon, is sometimes seen.

Streptococcal conjunctivitis with mild pseudo or severe true membrane formation may develop. The latter is characterized by a coagulative fibrinous exudate, penetrating the epithelial and subepithelial tissues. The conjunctivitis is similar to that caused by *C. diphtheriae*, except that the bulbar as well as the palpebral conjunctiva is involved (Plate VI, 1). The process may be complicated by rapid necrosis of the cornea, and perforation. Surprisingly, primary hypopyon keratitis due to *Streptococcus pyogenes* is rare.[37] Streptococcal conjunctivitis of endogenous origin seldom occurs. This is usually a mild pseudomembranous type which may persist for years or recur. The conjunctival culture is usually negative.

Uveitis, iritis, and iridocyclitis, often resulting from streptococcal focal infections, are possibly allergic in nature.

In all of these severe ocular conditions, *Streptococcus pyogenes* is chiefly responsible. However, the role of *Streptococcus mitis* must be mentioned. Although the distinction between the hemolysis of alpha and beta streptococci is more quantitative than qualitative (Wilson and Miles), in practice this division is still recognized.

Streptococcus mitis is not uncommonly a member of the normal flora. It can cause chronic focal infection and, in fact, does so more often than *Streptococcus pyogenes*. As a result, *Streptococcus mitis* may be responsible for most streptococcal hypersensitivity. Serologically and biochemically, only a few strains of alpha streptococci are defined.

A great similarity in culture and appearance exists between *Streptococcus mitis* and the pneumococcus, except that the latter is encapsulated (Plate V, 4, 5). For more details, see page 21.

Both organisms produce similar eye infections, and both respond well to the same therapy. The infections are manifested as acute catarrhal conjunctivitis, hypopyon keratitis, chronic dacryocystitis, or postoperative infection (Plate V, 1, 2).

Streptococcus salivarius is usually considered nonpathogenic. Morphologically it is similar to staphylococci and pathogenic streptococci. The most important identification is on the basis of cultural characteristics. *Streptococcus salivarius* grows luxuriantly on ordinary media and does not produce hemolysis.

The other streptococci, such as enterococci, are frequently the cause of urinary tract infections but rarely of ocular diseases.

Treatment.   Practically all streptococci are susceptible to sulfonamides and penicillin. No significant resistance of streptococci to penicillin is yet known. Sulfadiazine has been found highly effective in group A hemolytic streptococcal infections. However, exquisite sensitivity of a host to penicillin is not uncommon. Consequently, care must be taken when penicillin is given by parenteral injection.

The Pneumococcus
(Diplococcus pneumoniae)

Pneumococci are common inhabitants of the upper respiratory tract and are the primary cause of over 80 per cent of lobar pneumonia cases. The organisms were recognized by Pasteur in 1881, and in 1886 Fränkel and Weichselbaum described the pneumococcus as the agent of pneumonia. Before sulfonamides and antibiotics, the mortality from pneumococcal pneumonia was high.

Various studies have indicated that *Diplococcus pneumoniae* occurs frequently (40 to 70 per cent) in the normal conjunctival flora and naso-lacrimal system.

D. pneumoniae causes severe and serious ocular diseases. Because pneumococci are often present in normal flora, any ocular injury may lead to severe purulent infection, the most frequent being a hypopyon keratitis.

Morphology. *Diplococcus pneumoniae* is a species of the family *Lactobacillaceae*, tribe *Streptococceae*. The organisms are gram-positive, lancet-shaped, and occur in pairs. The diplococcal arrangement is found in clinical material and in smears from colonies grown on solid media. In fluid media, the cells occur chiefly in short chains (in contrast to the long chains of streptococci). Pneumococci can be decolorized very easily, showing some gram-negative forms, particularly in aged or very young cultures. The majority of pneumococci possess a polysaccharide capsule. This results in the appearance of smooth colonies. However, in any culture of pneumococci, a few nonencapsulated variants may occur, giving rise to rough colonies.

Culture. The pneumococcus does not grow on the usual media; it requires an enriched medium.

On blood agar plates, almost all ophthalmologic pneumococci appear as small, flat, shiny colonies surrounded by a green zone of incomplete alpha hemolysis (Plate IV, 4). The easily recognized green appearance is the most characteristic feature. Nevertheless these colonies may be confused with *Streptococcus mitis*.

Differential diagnosis between pneumococci and alpha streptococci can be made as follows: pneumococci are usually encapsulated; alpha streptococci are nonencapsulated. The bile solubility test, optochin sensitivity test (Plate IV, 3), and inulin fermentation are positive for pneumococci, negative for alpha streptococci.

Antigenic Structure. Cooper and other workers identified 32 serologic types of pneumococci; at present, there are known to be at least 75 or more. In ocular diseases, Types I, II, and III are most common. For serologic differentiation, two components are important. One is a polysaccharide (type-specific) present in the capsular material. Capsular polysaccharides determine both virulence and type of pneumococcus. It has been shown that antibodies against the pneumococcus are induced by capsular material and are type-specific. The other is a protein (group-specific) found in the somatic portion of the pneumococcus.

Immunity to pneumococcal infection is unfortunately incomplete and of brief duration only.

PNEUMOCOCCUS TYPING.   When pneumococci are mixed with type-specific rabbit antiserum, swelling of the capsule develops (Neufeld or Quellung reaction). The technic is simple: a loopful of undiluted antiserum is mixed with the specimen on the slide and covered. Then a loopful of Löffler's alkaline methylene blue is added at the margin of the coverglass. The capsule can also be demonstrated by a different method of staining—Hiss copper sulfate method, described on page 220 (Plate IV, 1).

Intraperitoneal inoculation of white mice is the most rapid method of obtaining a pure culture of pneumococci from contaminated material. It also determines the pathogenicity and demonstrates the capsule.

Pathogenicity and Pathology.   Pneumococci do not produce toxins. The disease process is due to invasiveness and multiplication of the bacteria. Nevertheless, the capsular polysaccharides are the determining factor in the virulence of the pneumococci and in the development of the disease. Besides, the capsule itself delays or prevents ingestion of pneumococci by phagocytosis. Predisposing factors, such as intercurrent infections, alcoholic intoxication, or debility, are sometimes more important in development of pneumococcal infection than is the virulence of the agent.

The characteristic pathology of pneumococcal infections is marked edema and fibrinous exudate. Both the onset and determination of the infection are sudden. The role of allergy in pneumococcal infection has been neglected (Smith and Conant). The sudden explosive onset of pneumococcal infection suggests an allergic reaction in individuals previously having pneumococcal infection. It occurs more often in adults than in children. Allergic reactions of the urticarial type may occur when convalescence begins.

Resistance.   Pneumococci are delicate organisms which die rapidly. They are readily killed by heat, 52° C requiring only 10 minutes. However, they often survive well at low temperatures, even at the freezing point.

Findings in the Eye.   The pneumococcus may cause a destructive hypopyon keratitis, is often found in chronic dacryocystitis, and is a frequent cause of acute conjunctivitis. It does not ordinarily cause chronic conjunctivitis or blepharoconjunctivitis.

CONJUNCTIVITIS.   Epidemics of acute pneumococcal conjunctivitis have been described, and it is the most common type in many parts of the United States. The infection seems to be more prevalent in the colder months and in northern climates. Frequent association with a "cold in the head" (but not with pneumonia) is characteristic. The infection has a predilection for children. Pneumococcal conjunctivitis similar to the conjunctivitis caused by the

Koch-Weeks bacillus is usually of moderate severity with a mild muco-purulent exudation. However, pronounced redness of the bulbar conjunctiva, often associated with petechial hemorrhages, is seen, usually in the upper fornix (Plate III, 1). These are more marked in pneumococcal conjunctivitis than in that due to the Koch-Weeks bacillus and are probably bacterial allergic reactions. Chemosis of the bulbar conjunctiva and enlargement of the preauricular glands may occur in severe cases.

Follicle formation is not infrequent in children but quite rare in pneumococcal conjunctivitis of adults.

It should be pointed out that the clinical appearance of pneumococcal conjunctivitis seems to vary in different countries; the discharge may become abundant and purulent, and corneal involvement is frequent. This picture is also seen in mixed infection, particularly with staphylococci.

The disease is contagious, and in smear numerous typical diplococci are usually seen; the exudate smear suffices for diagnosis (Plate III, 5). The pneumococci disappear rapidly in the regressive stage and are replaced by *Corynebacterium xerosis* and staphylococci. Subsidence of the conjunctivitis, even without treatment, is characteristic and occurs rapidly.

Corneal complications are rare in the United States. If they do occur, they are usually in the form of marginal infiltrates which later break down, forming small ulcers. The condition is not severe and heals along with the conjunctivitis. During the conjunctivitis, a few punctate, staining lesions may be seen in the epithelial layer of the cornea.

PNEUMOCOCCAL ULCER (ULCUS SERPENS). The pneumococcus is the commonest cause of central corneal ulcer,[27, 37] particularly in countries where chronic infection of the nasal mucosa is frequent. This results in blockage of the lacrimal passage, and the lacrimal sac serves as a main reservoir for pneumococcal infection. It is more common among farmers, stone masons, coal miners, or debilitated persons. Pneumococci do not invade normal corneal epithelium; the portal of entry is usually through a corneal abrasion, generally caused by a foreign body.

This pneumococcal corneal ulcer is central and usually occurs as a primary entity without a preceding conjunctivitis; the ulcer is typically associated with sterile hypopyon. The hypopyon indicates an iritis or iridocyclitis due to toxic products. If the cornea is perforated, an infected hypopyon is likely. The clinical picture is characterized initially by a heavy infiltrate, yellowish in color, which rapidly breaks down, resulting in ulcer formation. The ulcer spreads on the surface of the cornea in a particular direction, hence the name serpiginous ulcer, or ulcus serpens of Saemisch (1870) is used (Duke-Elder, p. 1934). The spreading, or progressive, margin is usually undermined in pocketlike formation (Plate III, 2). The organisms are numerous there, and the scraping should be taken from this area. The typical morphology of pneumococci may be sufficient to be diagnostic in the scraping (Plate III, 6). Later, the ulceration extends more deeply, and perforation of the cornea often follows. Then the infection may become intra-ocular or even result in panophthalmitis.

Pneumococci are regarded by many authorities as the principal etiologic agent for central hypopyon ulcer. However, at Bellevue Hospital, *Moraxella lacunata* was found to be a more frequent causative agent.

CHRONIC DACRYOCYSTITIS. This almost always arises secondarily to obstruction or stenosis of the nasolacrimal duct. When free drainage through the duct is hindered, stasis of tears results and this is a favorable condition for infection. In the warm, dark lacrimal sac with its sufficient food, the bacteria grow as in an incubator. A large number of encapsulated pneumococci are most commonly found within it, along with other organisms. A lacrimal sac so affected becomes a constant source of infection for the eye, and while always dangerous, it is even more so when overlooked before intraocular surgery. Chronic dacryocystitis can easily be missed because there is little or no local inflammation. This has been called by Theodore "silent" dacryocystitis. In case of chronic unilateral conjunctivitis, chronic dacryocystitis must be first suggested. Examination of the nasolacrimal system before intraocular surgery is recommended, especially for older patients. The examination should include pressure over the lacrimal sac as well as irrigation.

The chronic process may suddenly exacerbate into acute dacryocystitis if the infection invades the perilacrimal tissue. Many factors, often unrecognizable, may play a role. If a lacrimal fistula develops (Plate III, 4) and is long existing, granulomatous masses resembling tumor may result (Plate III, 3).

Postoperative infections are often caused by pneumococci, and this organism is by far the most common pathogen for panophthalmitis following wounds of the eye. Presurgical examination of the tear sac is important.

Bacterial metastasis in pneumococcal septicemia has been found in the form of small, translucent nodules in the choroid or retina.

Treatment. Before the antibiotic era, optochin (ethylhydrocupreine hydrochloride) was regarded as specific treatment for pneumococcal infection. It can be given only locally, as it is highly toxic systemically. In superficial infections such as conjunctivitis, 1 per cent optochin solution is useful, especially in areas where antibiotics are difficult to obtain.

Of the bacterial infections to which man is subject, pneumococcal infection is the most susceptible to penicillin, tetracycline or other antibiotics, and sulfonamides. There are as yet no known forms of pneumococci resistant to antibiotics.

Antibiotics can be applied locally or systemically. In conjunctivitis, local therapy suffices. In cases of hypopyon ulcer both local and systemic administration of antibiotics is required. For the latter, the usual treatment is from 300,000 to 1,000,000 units of penicillin three times a day.

If dacryocystitis is present, immediate dacryocystectomy should be considered. Most attempts to treat central hypopyon ulcer in the presence of dacryocystitis have proved unsuccessful.

Proper care of the iris must not be forgotten.

THE CORYNEBACTERIUM GENUS

As the name implies, corynebacteria are clublike in form, this being due to the presence of Babes-Ernst metachromatic granules.

Included are the broad group of diphtheroids and *Corynebacterium diphtheriae*. Most diphtheroids are human parasites living mainly on the skin and mucous membranes. *Corynebacterium xerosis* is an almost constant saprophyte of the conjunctiva. While saprophytic for man, some diphtheroids are pathogenic for animals.

Of the entire group, only *C. diphtheriae* (the diphtheria bacillus) is an important human pathogen.

Corynebacterium diphtheriae

While no longer a serious problem in many areas, diphtheria was formerly a dread disease. Even today in areas where immunization is not practical, the infection is still a severe threat, especially for children.

Morphology. While this bacillus is gram-positive, the gram stain is of little value in studying its morphology. To demonstrate the metachromatic granules, a special stain such as Neisser's must be used (see page 220). Methylene blue is a good routine diagnostic stain. Diphtheria bacilli are large and slender, straight or slightly curved pleomorphic rods. The metachromatic granules are typically situated at the poles, the rod being a drumstick shape. The bacilli are arranged at various angles to one another, forming V, T, or L shapes, and groups of the organisms form clusters resembling Chinese letters; this appearance aids considerably in diagnosis (Plate VIII, 3). In smear from the culture, true branching may be seen.

Corynebacterium diphtheriae is divided into three subgroups: gravis, mitis, and intermedius, depending upon their grade of infectivity. The subgroups have much in common.

Culture. Diphtheria bacilli grow slowly on ordinary media. The best medium is Löffler's blood serum medium. Use of a routine blood agar plate is advisable for identification of other bacteria, especially hemolytic streptococci which may occur together with *C. diphtheriae*.

Colonies of *C. diphtheriae* on Löffler's medium are small, round, granular, moist, slightly creamy or gray, and have irregular edges (Plate VIII, 5).

Tellurite medium is used additionally to Löffler's blood serum medium to differentiate *C. diphtheriae* from the diphtheroid bacilli and to distinguish subgroups of *C. diphtheriae*. The colonies of *C. diphtheriae* are a distinct black due to reduction of tellurite (Plate VIII, 4A).

On blood agar, colonies are usually small, grayish, and granular. Beta-hemolysis may be slight or absent (Plate VIII, 4B).

In contrast to the slowly growing diphtheroids, the diphtheria bacilli grow rapidly, requiring only 6 to 12 hours of incubation.

In its biochemical reactions, *C. diphtheriae* produces acid (not gas) in glucose but not in sucrose (Plate IX, 4).

Toxin Production and Pathogenicity. *Corynebacterium diphtheriae* produces a powerful toxin but has little invasiveness; the bacteria hardly ever enter the blood stream. The toxin is the principal factor in establishing disease. It rapidly diffuses from the primary focus, chiefly tonsillitis, to other parts of the body, and toxemia may result.

The toxin stimulates formation of a powerful antitoxin which imparts prolonged immunity. Antiserum containing powerful antibodies, which is important for treatment, is prepared by repeated injection of purified toxoid into various animals, such as rabbits, guinea pigs, horses, and sheep.

Pathology. Diphtheria bacilli cause a local infection of the mucous membranes, particularly the pharynx and more rarely the conjunctiva. The epithelium becomes necrotic from absorbed toxin and is embedded in a massive fibropurulent exudate, forming a pseudomembrane. If subepithelial tissue is involved, a true membrane develops. The capillaries enter the membrane, and therefore bleeding occurs if one attempts to remove it. The bacilli multiply in this tissue, and their toxin is rapidly absorbed. It may damage distant parts of the body, causing parenchymatous degeneration, fatty infiltration, necrosis, or gross hemorrhages. The toxin often damages the nerves, resulting in paralysis, and the eye may be involved.

Findings in the Eye. *C. diphtheriae* is a primary cause of conjunctivitis, although this is now rare. Depending upon the severity of the process, two clinical types of conjunctivitis are distinguished: pseudomembranous and true membranous. Both usually follow pharyngeal diphtheria in children aged 2 to 8. The pseudomembrane may be removed without occurrence of bleeding, whereas removal of a true membrane leads to bleeding. In the latter, the entire conjunctival tissue to the tarsal plate may be penetrated by a thick network of fibrin (Plate VIII, 1) and the vessels obliterated by thrombosis.

Three stages are characteristic in the severe membranous conjunctivitis:

1. Infiltrated or indurated stage: the lids and conjunctiva become almost impossible to evert. Pressure from the tense indurated lids may cause corneal damage, even necrosis.

2. Suppurative stage: the lids soften, the membrane separates, and underlying granulation may be seen.

3. Cicatrization stage: scarring of the lid conjunctiva is seen.

Diphtheritic infections may be complicated by other bacterial invaders, including staphylococci, pneumococci, and streptococci. The latter severely aggravate the process.

The *C. diphtheriae* cells usually disappear by the time the membrane is gone, but some persons become chronic carriers.

Diphtheritic mucopurulent conjunctivitis, indistinguishable from other bacterial conjunctivitides, may also be seen (Plate VIII, 2). Conjunctivitis due to *C. diphtheriae* is rare in the United States; when it occurs it is almost always the pseudomembranous type. It is rarely associated with pharyngeal diphtheria, and there may or may not be systemic symptoms. Active immunization of children by diphtheria toxoid is not permanent; hence the disease may occur in previously immunized adults.

Corneal involvement may be due directly to toxin, to pressure as mentioned before, and to the decrease of corneal nutrition resulting from thrombosis of limbal capillaries. The typically necrotic diphtheritic keratitis may become purulent due to secondary infection. Ulceration and perforation of the cornea may result.

Palsy of extraocular muscles or, more frequently, paralysis of accommodation may occur. The latter is usually permanent.

Diagnosis. There are no differential diagnostic indications in the clinical picture of conjunctivitis. Diagnosis depends almost entirely on bacteriologic examination, a problem involving delay. The bacteriologist with long experience may obtain a rapid preliminary diagnosis by direct, specially stained smear. Otherwise, the diagnosis requires several days of special study. This must be confirmed by cultural identification of the organism and by the virulence test.

VIRULENCE TEST. This can be done in different ways. The most definitive type of testing is by intracutaneous or cutaneous inoculation of a bacterial suspension into guinea pigs or rabbits. This test is not practical from a clinical standpoint as it takes much time and is quite costly. For these reasons, the in vitro test is recommended.

In vitro test (Jawetz et al.).[15] "A strip of filter paper, saturated with antitoxin, is placed on an agar plate containing 20 per cent horse serum. The cultures to be tested for toxigenicity are streaked across the plate at right angles to the filter paper. After 48 hours incubation, the antitoxin diffusion from the paper strip has precipitated the toxin diffusion from the toxigenic cultures in lines radiating from the intersection of the streak of bacterial growth" (Plate IX, 2). This test is best done in a general bacteriology laboratory. If the ophthalmologist suspects diphtheria, he should immediately send material to the bacteriology laboratory.

Treatment. Antidiphtheric serum therapy is specific. Antitoxin should be given as soon as the diagnosis is made. In severe cases, intravenous injection of large doses (4,000 or 6,000 or 10,000 units) is necessary. Usually one injection is enough, but if necessary it can be repeated in 10 to 12 hours to avoid anaphylactic reaction. In mild cases 2,000 units intramuscularly may be satisfactory. Antibiotics topically and warm compresses are required. If membranes are present, avoid silver nitrate.

To prevent secondary infection, such antibiotics as penicillin, strepto-mycin, tetracycline, or erythromycin may be needed.

Corynebacterium xerosis

C. xerosis alone of the numerous diphtheroids is considered a strictly ophthalmic bacterium. It has not been found on any other organ than the conjunctiva, and it is almost constantly present there. It grows as a sapro-phyte, usually on desquamating conjunctival epithelium. This bacillus has never been shown to be pathogenic for the eye. However, its pathogenicity has been shown in experiments.[40] It should not be forgotten that some diphtheroids can be pathogenic for animals. It often confuses laboratory diagnosis because of morphologic characteristics similar to those of other bacteria.

Morphology.   The bacilli are short, thick, curved, and gram-positive, with very irregular size and shape. Metachromatic granules are generally distributed throughout the whole bacillus, giving it a barred appearance (Plate VII, 6). The organisms are frequently seen in clumps or arranged at angles giving V, L, and T formations, or in palisades. In smear, C. xerosis may be confused with the pneumococcus if the metachromatic granules are isolated at the poles, thus giving intensive bipolar staining. At other times, the bacillus may have a beaded form and thus be confused with strepto-cocci. Most important for the identification of this organism is the irregu-larity of its size and shape, and even when there are V or L forms, one bacillus tends to be of different size and shape from the other (Plate VII, 1, 2).

C. xerosis differs from C. diphtheriae by being shorter, thicker, and more clumped and curved. Usually the metachromatic granules are not at the end of the organism but are distributed throughout its whole body.

Culture.   C. xerosis grows much more slowly than C. diphtheriae, sometimes taking a few days to a week, averaging 48 hours. Colonies on blood agar are tiny, dustlike, gray, opaque, dull, and dry looking (Plate VII, 5). They adhere firmly to the medium and do not emulsify easily. On Löffler's serum, they grow faster though not as quickly as C. diphtheriae, and the colonies are smaller and drier.

C. xerosis produces acid in glucose and sucrose.

Findings in the Eye.   C. xerosis is not a pathogen but rather a normal inhabitant of the conjunctiva. The bacilli may appear in large numbers in any infectious conjunctivitis, especially during the period of convalescence. In some infections they are present throughout the course, because of a symbiotic relationship with etiologic bacteria, such as Moraxella lacunata. A large number of C. xerosis cells may be found in vitamin A deficiency be-cause of the marked "keratinization" of the conjunctival epithelium. Scrap-ing from Bitot's spot (Plate VII, 3) shows the amount of the organisms to be similar to that in a smear from pure culture.

A large number of cells of *C. xerosis* are invariably present in kerato-malacia. This condition, with complete destruction of the cornea, occurs usually in children with debility and malnutrition (Plate VII, 4).

SPOREFORMING BACILLI

AEROBIC SPOREFORMING BACILLI

To this group belong a large number of saprophytic strains, including *Bacillus subtilis*. They are inhabitants of soil, water, air, and vegetation. *B. anthracis* is the only pathogenic species of this genus.

Bacillus anthracis

Anthrax was known even in antiquity. It was the first disease of proven bacterial origin. The disease is still widespread, occurring in every country, although it is prevalent only in certain areas. In the United States about 50 cases of anthrax are reported every year.

Morphology. These bacilli are large, square-ended, gram-positive organisms, usually arranged in long chains. Their spores are situated at about the center of the organism. The bacilli are nonmotile. In the specimen, they may be so few as to escape finding under the microscope. Culture of the patient's blood, or a specimen from the lesion, or both, are necessary.

Cultivation. *B. anthracis* is aerobic (or facultatively anaerobic) and grows well on nutrient agar and other general media. Blood agar is used to differentiate the hemolytic properties of *B. anthracis* from the known hemolytic saprophytic strains of the species. However, the test for pathogenicity is essential. The colonies appear round, with a cut-glass appearance. A membranous consistency of the colonies is due to the formation of parallel chains by the bacilli.

Pathogenicity and Pathology. *B. anthracis* is pathogenic for man and most animals. Grazing animals, such as sheep and cattle, are more commonly affected. Man may be infected by contact with the wool, hair, or hide of diseased animals. Anthrax is primarily a disease of the skin, affecting especially such exposed areas as the head and neck. Infection follows injury to the skin. The bacilli spread via lymphatics to the bloodstream and multiply rapidly.[18] If untreated, the disease is usually followed by septicemia and death.

Findings in the Eye. Anthrax of the lid occurs but is extremely rare. The manifestations are similar to anthrax infections of other parts of the body. Two clinical forms occur: 1, malignant pustule and 2, malignant edema. The site of a malignant pustule can be on either lid. It begins in the form of a pimple, followed by a vesicle, then by a pustule, and finally an ulcer or gangrene. The lesion is not painful, and the regional lymph glands are only mildly involved. Large areas may be involved, and heavy scarring is a sequela. The process may extend to involve the cornea and other parts of the eye. Ulceration of the cornea, panophthalmitis, and exophthalmos with optic atrophy may occur.

Malignant edema of the lid is characterized by marked edema with the skin showing little or no inflammation. These cases are more difficult to diagnose, and septicemia is more likely to occur in this form of anthrax.

Treatment. Most antibiotics are effective against anthrax bacilli. Treatment must be started early to prevent development of a toxic process. Antisera and antibiotics considerably reduce mortality.

Bacillus subtilis

This bacillus lives in dust, milk, soil, and particularly hay. Hence, a well-known synonym for the bacillus is the hay bacillus. Morphologically it is similar to *B. anthracis*. It grows freely on all general media and is often a laboratory contaminant. The colonies appear granular, are usually adherent to the media, and may cause hemolysis. While not considered pathogenic, if introduced into the vitreous body, which is supposed to be an excellent medium for *B. subtilis*, it can cause a panophthalmitis. Unique cases of iridocyclitis, postoperative panophthalmitis, and ring abscess of the cornea due to *B. subtilis* have been described.

ANAEROBIC SPOREFORMING BACILLI

The Clostridia

A number of species belong to the genus, *Clostridium*. They are distributed in soil or in the intestinal tract of man and animals. They become pathogenic in injured tissue, producing toxin and rapid putrefaction of protein. The most common pathogenic strains for man are *Clostridium botulinum, Cl. tetani*, and *Cl. perfringens*.

Morphologically, all are bacilli with a drumstick appearance. Bulging of the wall at one end of the rod is caused by spores. All are gram-positive. While the organism arrangement varies, it is often in long chains.

Cultivation is difficult, since the bacilli of this genus are strictly anaerobic. It is best to have these specimens examined by a general bacteriologist.

Ocular infections caused by these species are rare, and literature on the subject is limited. Gas gangrene of the lids, eyeball (panophthalmitis), or orbit may develop following injury and contact with contaminated soil or manure. In these cases air bubbles can be seen.[21] A violent infection often associated with other organisms, especially streptococci, may occur. Except for gas gangrene, other clostridial eye infections are only secondary to the systemic diseases. Tsutsui, however, has reported a case of primary tetanus infection of the cornea.

Treatment. Since in clostridial infections toxin is the factor establishing the process, antitoxin must be used. It is usually polyvalent, containing antibodies to several toxins, and it should be administered as soon as possible. The antitoxin can be used together with antibiotics.

THE MYCOBACTERIA

This group is comprised of acid-fast bacilli, the majority of which are saprophytic. Only *Mycobacterium tuberculosis* and *M. leprae* are known pathogens for man. Both are intracellular parasites which cause a chronic granulomatous process.

Mycobacterium tuberculosis

There are four variants of *M. tuberculosis:* var. *hominus,* var. *bovis,* var. *avian,* and var. *muris.* Man is affected only by the first two types. Both are equally pathogenic for man by either the respiratory or the gastrointestinal route. The most common variant is *hominus,* which invades the body by being inhaled or ingested, or directly through the skin or mucous membranes.

The location and pattern of the tuberculosis lesions indicate the route of primary infection. If invasion is by inhalation, tuberculosis of the lungs develops. Scrofula or cervical adenitis results from ingestion. Entrance through the skin or mucous membranes is usually followed by arid ulcers with marked enlargement of the regional lymph nodes. An example is oculoglandular Parinaud's syndrome in primary tuberculosis of the conjunctiva.

Morphology. In smear, the acid-fast tubercle bacilli are fairly long, straight, curved, or bent. With Ziehl-Neelsen stain (page 219) they appear irregularly red with a granular or beaded appearance. They may occur singly or in groups. If the organisms are arranged at angles to each other, they resemble corynebacteria. Their appearances are so characteristic that identification can usually be made by microscopic examination of a direct smear (Plate X, 4).

In animal tissue, the bacilli are more regular, longer, and thinner. In culture, there is pleomorphism with coccoid, club-shaped, filamentous, or even branching forms.

Tubercle bacilli take the gram stain poorly and hence are not classified by this method but rather by acid-fast staining. The simplest and most commonly used stain is Ziehl-Neelsen's. Numerous other staining methods, including fluorescent microscopy, have been utilized.

Culture. Cultivation of tubercle bacilli is a difficult and prolonged procedure. They are strictly aerobic (probably the chief basis for the success of lung collapse therapy). A variety of complicated media have been used to grow the bacilli. Löwenstein's medium is supposed to be more satisfactory for both the human and bovine types (Plate X, 5). On this medium, the colonies are creamy, dull, rough, and granular. Incubation requires at least two months.

Chemical Composition.   Tubercle bacilli contain lipids in the highest percentage and proteins (largely nucleoproteins) which are responsible for tuberculin sensitivity. The bacilli also contain a relatively small amount of polysaccharides which can induce an anaphylactic type of hypersensitivity.

Pathology.   The pathology is determined by the virulence and number of tubercle bacilli. Resistance and hypersensitivity of the host are even more important. Two types of lesions are produced. One is the exudative acute inflammatory type, which can either be absorbed or result in massive necrosis. This process in the lungs is similar to bacterial pneumonia. The other is a productive type characterized by a chronic granuloma or tubercle. The tubercle consists of a central zone in which are found typical Langhans' giant cells and mononuclear epithelioid cells. The central zone is surrounded by a cuff of lymphocytes. Dead tissue at the center of the tubercle becomes cheesy (caseated); this may be followed by a cavity or fibrosis and calcification. The tubercle bacilli are found intracellularly in monocytes, giant cells, or reticuloendothelial cells. The bacilli may spread from the initial site via lymphatics and the blood stream to all organs, causing miliary tuberculosis. (If the spread is via lymphatics, the regional glands are first involved.)

Tuberculin Diagnostic Methods.   Tuberculin is an extract of tubercle bacilli or a filtrate of a broth culture. Koch, using tuberculin for subcutaneous injections, produced a local inflammation in tuberculous animals, followed by necrosis, without any increase in their original infections. This has since been known as Koch's phenomenon, a state of hypersensitivity induced by previous exposure to tubercle bacilli. The reaction is negative in normal animals. Hence, Koch's phenomenon is an important diagnostic indication.

There are now available various kinds of tuberculins for diagnostic or therapeutic purposes. The best known are Koch's original tuberculin, known as Old Tuberculin (OT), and Seibert's purified protein derivate (PPD).

Several tuberculin diagnostic tests have been devised: the Mantoux intracutaneous test, the Pirquet cutaneous test, and the Vollmer patch test. The Mantoux test is the most popular because it is the most accurate and gives quantitative measurement. Koch's original subcutaneous injection is now used only in veterinary practice. We refer you to the table, Dilutions of Tuberculin, in Smith and Conant, page 344.

Some individuals, particularly Negroes or patients with tuberculous eye diseases, may be extremely sensitive to tuberculin. Therefore, an initial dose must be done with caution.

These tuberculin tests are of value in young children; even so, a positive test does not indicate present active disease, only past infection. It may be negative if the tuberculous infection is superimposed by measles or Boeck's sarcoid.

Findings in the Eye. Tuberculous diseases of the eye are rare.[38] The tuberculous allergic manifestation is more common than infection due to tubercle bacilli themselves.

Phlyctenules of the conjunctiva and cornea are the commonest manifestations of tuberculous allergy, especially in the glandular type of tuberculosis. Phlyctenulosis is still a common disease of childhood, particularly in Arctic regions [12] and underdeveloped countries. It is usually associated with enlargement of the tonsils and adenoids, swelling of the cervical lymphatic glands, eczema, and catarrh of various mucosa. In some countries it is still a principal cause of blindness. There are several clinical entities of phlyctenules, with common symptoms such as severe photophobia and blepharospasmus, itching, and often secondary bacterial infection, particularly staphylococcal.

PHLYCTENULAR CONJUNCTIVITIS. The limbus is a site of phlyctenules. They are gray or pinkish white elevations vascularized on the periphery; they ulcerate easily. They are often multiple miliary elevations (Plate XI, 1), sometimes involving the entire limbal area. Ring ulcer may result. Ulceration of the phlyctenules is the basic feature which differentiates them from other circumscribed lesions of the limbus, such as the limbal form of vernal conjunctivitis, rosacea, and pinguecula. The process usually heals without a trace but tends to recur.

PHLYCTENULAR KERATITIS. The phlyctenules are situated predominantly in the exposed area of the cornea, either peripherally or centrally. They represent vascular or avascular circumscribed lesions having a tendency to necrotize with resulting deep ulceration. Perforation may occur. In undernourished children the keratitis may become pustular and perforated (Plate XI, 3), due to secondary bacterial invasion, particularly staphylococcal. Leukoma adhaerens, anterior staphyloma, and blindness are the consequences. In less severe keratitis, single or multiple maculae remain and, if central, decrease vision.

Fascicular keratitis is manifested by a migrating phlyctenule pulling a vascular tail along the surface of the cornea. The movement can start at the limbus, moving toward the center, or it may cross the entire cornea in the form of a narrow, vascular ribbon (Plate XI, 2).

Phlyctenular (eczematous, scrofulous) pannus, unlike trachomatous pannus, may develop in any peripheral part of the cornea, mainly the lower, and in a late state of phlyctenules (Plate XI, 4).

Tubercle bacilli have not been demonstrated in any phlyctenular disease. In a scraping from the involved area, eosinophils may be present.

External eye infections due to tubercle bacilli themselves are rare. They usually develop secondarily, either by contiguity or by metastasis from other parts of the body. Occasionally, tuberculosis of the eye can be primary.

LUPUS VULGARIS. The process is the most common type of skin tuberculosis. The lid skin, conjunctiva, cornea, and lacrimal sac can be involved by continuation from adjacent tissue. Tuberculous ulcers of the lid margin resembling carcinoma, or nodules resembling chalazion, may occur.

CHRONIC DACRYOCYSTITIS. In young children, particularly girls, this is often a continuation of adjacent bone tuberculosis, or it can be primary.

TUBERCULOUS DACRYOADENITIS AND TUBERCULOSIS OF THE ORBITAL BONE. Both are usually of metastatic origin, are painless, with mild inflammatory reactions, and in the later stage, are characterized by fistula.

In all these processes, the finding of tubercle bacilli may often help establish the diagnosis.

KERATITIS DUE TO M. TUBERCULOSIS. Tuberculous infection of the cornea is mainly of metastatic origin. The resultant type of keratitis is typically deep nodular and may be abscesslike, often involving the upper external quadrant (Plate X, 2) (as seen also in leprotic keratitis). The process is usually unilateral. As the cornea is a poor culture medium for the tubercle bacilli, the latter are very rarely found in tuberculous keratitis, and diagnosis is thus based mainly on the typical clinical picture. However, this type of keratitis could be an allergic manifestation. One also finds a diffuse interstitial keratitis, which is probably an anaphylactic phenomenon.

PRIMARY TUBERCULOSIS OF THE CONJUNCTIVA. This usually occurs in the palpebral conjunctiva. It is of exogenous origin, due to direct invasion by the tubercle bacilli. A few clinical types are distinguished: ulcerative, hyperplastic, and mixed. The hyperplastic variety is subdivided into nodular and papillary types. The nodules appear as yellowish gray granules resembling those of trachoma. In the papillary type, the papillae may become pedunculated, and ulcers usually develop on the tops of the papillae (Plate X, 1). A polypoidal type, or tuberculoma, has been described.

Primary tuberculosis of the lacrimal sac is recorded.

The common characteristics of the above types are: the finding of tubercle bacilli in scrapings or histologic sections and an oculoglandular Parinaud's syndrome (swelling of the regional lymph glands).

The uveal tract and retina may be involved, usually in adults.

When tuberculosis of the inner eye is suspected careful tuberculin testing must be used to avoid hypersensitivity reactions which can be dangerous for the eye.

Treatment. Combined treatment with streptomycin, para-aminosalicylic acid (PAS), and isonicotinic acid hydrazide (INH) greatly reduces mortality but does not prevent the infections. In metastatic ocular tuberculosis, systemic treatment is required; this may also be indicated for primary ocular tuberculosis. The usual topical treatment for keratitis or iritis must be added. In allergic manifestations, the effect of cortisone can be prompt. Since resistance and hypersensitivity are decisive in tuberculous diseases, care of the general health may be even more important than the drug treatment. This includes proper diet, good hygiene, fresh air, sufficient rest, and other factors.

Mycobacterium leprae

The ancient, still dreaded disease, leprosy, is also called Hansen's disease, after Gerhard Hansen who in 1874 reported his discovery of M. leprae.

Endemic areas of leprosy are found in most parts of the world. However, it is fairly common in tropical and subtropical regions.

Leprosy is a slowly progressive, chronic granulomatous disease affecting skin, mucous membranes, peripheral nerves, and usually the lymph nodes. The portal of entry is probably the skin and nasal mucosa. The incubation period is of indefinite length, from two weeks to many years. Children are most sensitive to the infection but seldom develop symptoms of leprosy until adulthood. Since the mode of transmission is uncertain, segregation of infected persons in leprosaria is still practiced. As a prophylactic measure, it is recommended that children be segregated from their leprous parents.

Morphology. The bacilli are pleomorphic and acid-fast, resembling tubercle bacilli. Morphologically they resemble diphtheroids, varying in size, and in shape from long, straight, or curved to irregular coccoid or granular forms (Plate XII, 4). They decolorize more readily (by Ziehl-Neelsen) than tubercle bacilli and are arranged in clumps, bundles, palisades, or globular masses. The organisms are regularly found in scrapings, especially in the nodular form of leprosy. They grow best intracellularly in endothelial and mononuclear cells. The role of the bacillus as sole etiologic agent is not completely established. The bacilli have never been cultivated and leprosy has never been reproduced experimentally.

Serologic tests are of no value.

Pathology. Leprosy is characterized by the production of leproma (granuloma), diffuse infiltration, or both. Pathologic examination reveals connective tissue cells, many plasma cells, and a conglomerate of lepra cells (large, irregular, poorly defined masses) loaded with bacilli (in the nodular form). The cells probably are degenerated giant cells.

Clinical Features. Clinical manifestations of leprosy vary greatly. The clinical symptoms may differ even in the same geographic area, or they can be common in different clinical forms of leprosy. Therefore, several clinical or pathologic divisions have been proposed. In practice, two divisions are most acceptable: the nodular form and the neural anesthetic form (also called maculo-anesthetic); both can be present in the same patient. In the nodular type, lesions appear on the exposed skin surfaces, i.e., hands and face, especially on the nose (Plate XII, 2), forehead, and lips (causing the characteristic lionlike facies). This is a contagious form, and bacilli are constantly found.

The neural (maculo-anesthetic) form is characterized by diffuse infiltration of peripheral nerves (chronic interstitial neuritis), with consequent loss of sensation. Therefore the hands and feet are easily damaged, often with resultant grotesque deformation. Clawlike appearance of the hands (Plate

XII, 6) may develop because of nerve and muscle atrophy. The cell response is the same as in the nodular form, except that bacilli are very few and are difficult to find.

Findings in the Eye. Leprosy may involve any or all of the ocular structures. The incidence of ocular involvement may be 75 to 90 per cent. [10,13,17]

Corneal involvement is common [2] and is the main cause of blindness in lepers. Three main clinical forms of leprotic keratitis are distinguished: 1, leprotic superficial punctate keratitis; 2, leprotic pannus in the upper half, similar to trachomatous (or in the outer quadrant of the cornea); and 3, interstitial keratitis. These forms may represent one process in its different stages. The common characteristics of the three are: corneal anesthesia, thickening of the nerves in the stroma, scattered, chalky, minute grains (Plate XII, 1), the presence of the organisms, and no tendency to ulceration. Sometimes, a very destructive process in the form of a tumorlike leproma invades and destroys the entire cornea. Corneal leproma (Plate XII, 5) shows a yellowish mass with deep vascularization; the process is indolent and symptomless, resembling an old scar. The nodules may show central necrosis, which sometimes results in the formation of ulcer, perforation, and staphyloma.

The lids are frequently affected. The nodular type of leprosy may typically involve the skin of the upper lids but usually spares the lower lid and lid margins. However, in the area adjacent to the nodules, the lashes fall out.

The conjunctiva is rarely affected. In nodular leprosy, miliary, yellowish, or white nodules develop, usually at the upper outer quadrant of the limbus, more rarely in the bulbar conjunctiva. The nodules may ulcerate, and the process often spreads into the cornea and the sclera.

Paralysis of the orbicularis muscle may occur in neural maculo-anesthetic leprosy; ulcerative keratitis, papillary conjunctivitis, and fleshy pterygium may result, secondary to the lagophthalmos.

Leprosy predominantly involves the anterior segment of the eye. However, the posterior segment may be affected, and according to Pendergast, fundus changes took place in 42 out of 241 patients. The case illustrated showed a group of discrete lesions in the periphery of the fundus (Plate XII, 3) resembling the picture reported by Trantas. Elliott reported six cases of retinal pearls visible through the ophthalmoscope. There have been described superficial nodules in the retina. Granulomatous uveitis, with tissue necrosis and enormous numbers of bacilli, has been recorded.

Treatment. No specific treatment is known. It is extremely important to pay attention to the general health. Antituberculosis treatment may have some effect; the use of streptomycin or the sulfones Promin and Diasone has been reported as helpful. A long period of treatment, from two to nine years, is required.

REFERENCES

1. Allen, J. H. Experimental production of conjunctivitis with staphylococci, Am. J. Ophth., 22:1218, 1939.
2. ——— and Byers, J. L. The pathology of ocular leprosy. 1. The cornea, Arch. Ophth., 64:216, 1960.
3. Arouh, H., Zambrano, J., and Lis, M. Ocular manifestation in botulism (abstract), Am. J. Ophth., 38:282, 1954.
4. Berens, C., and Nilson, E. L. Relationship between the bacteriology of the conjunctiva and nasal mucosa, Am. J. Ophth., 27:747, 1944.
5. Brown, J. H. The use of blood agar for the study of streptococci, The Rockefeller Institute for Medical Research (Monograph 9), 1919, 122 pp.
6. Burns, R. P. Postoperative infections in an ophthalmic hospital, Am. J. Ophth., 48:519, 1959.
7. Chace, R. R., and Locatcher-Khorazo, D. Keratoconjunctivitis due to a diphtheroid-like organism, Arch. Ophth., 37:497, 1947.
8. Cooper, G., et al. The further separation of types among the pneumococci hitherto included in group IV and the development of therapeutic antisera for these types, J. Exper. Med., 55:531, 1932.
9. Davenport, R., and Smith, C. Panophthalmitis due to an organism of the *Bacillus subtilis* group, Brit. J. Ophth., 36:389, 1952.
10. Elliot, D. C. Leprosy, a disease of childhood: with special reference to early findings in the eye, ear, nose and throat of children examined at the national leprosarium at Carville, Louisiana, J. Pediat., 35:189, 1949.
11. Fränkel, A. Bakteriologische mittheilungen, Ztschr. klin. Med., 10:426, 1886.
12. Fritz, M. H., Thygeson, P., and Durham, D. G. Phlyctenular keratoconjunctivitis among Alaskan natives, Am. J. Ophth., 34:177, 1951.
13. Harley, R. D. Ocular leprosy in Panama, Am. J. Ophth., 29:295, 1946.
14. Holmes, W. J. Leprosy of the eye, Tr. Am. Ophth. Soc., 55:145, 1957.
15. Jawetz, E., Melnick, J. L., and Adelberg, E. A. Review of Medical Microbiology, 5th ed., Los Altos, California, Lange Medical Publications, 1962.
16. Julianelle, L. A., Boots, R. H., and Harrison, G. H. The treatment of staphylococcal infections of the eye by immunization with toxoid, Am. J. Ophth., 25:431, 1942.
17. Kennedy, P. J. Ocular manifestations in leprosy, Am. J. Ophth., 35:1360, 1952.
18. Krauss, F., and Spikes, N. O. Edematous anthrax of the face resulting in meningitis, Am. J. Ophth., 9:337, 1926.
19. Kronenberg, B. A case of multiple tuberculous nodules of the episclera, Am. J. Ophth., 29:86, 1946.
20. Lancefield, R. C. A serological differentiation of human and other groups of hemolytic streptococci, J. Exper. Med., 57:571, 1933.
21. Leavelle, R. B. Gas gangrene panophthalmitis, Arch. Ophth., 53:634, 1955.
22. Locatcher-Khorazo, D., and Gutierrez, E. Bacteriophage typing of *Staphylococcus aureus*, Arch. Ophth., 63:774, 1960.
23. Pasteur, L. Bull. Acad. nat. méd., 10(2me série): 76, 1881.
24. Pendergast, J. J. Ocular leprosy in the United States, Arch. Ophth., 23:112, 1940.
25. Raymond, L. F. Staphylococcus sensitivity in chorioretinitis, Am. J. Ophth., 48:846, 1959.
26. Ré, B. V., and Muhlmann, V. Primary diphtheritic conjunctivitis in the new-born (abstract), Am. J. Ophth., 25:1130, 1942.
27. Rhodes, A. J. Studies on the bacteriology of hypopyon ulcer, Brit. J. Ophth., 23:627, 1939.
28. Scobee, R. G. The role of the meibomian glands in recurrent conjunctivitis, Am. J. Ophth., 25:184, 1942.
29. Suie, T., and Taylor, F. W. Incidence of coagulase-positive staphylococci in external ocular infections, Arch. Ophth., 53:706, 1955.

30. Theodore, F. H., and Schlossman, A.   Ocular Allergy, Baltimore, Williams & Wilkins Co., 1958.
31. ——— "Silent" dacryocystitis, Arch. Ophth., 40:157, 1948.
32. Thygeson, P.   Treatment of staphylococcic blepharoconjunctivitis with staphylococcus toxoid, Arch. Ophth., 26:430, 1941.
33. ——— Etiology and treatment of blepharitis, Arch. Ophth., 36:445, 1946.
34. ——— Observations on non-tuberculous phlyctenuclar keratoconjunctivitis, Tr. Am. Acad. Ophth., 58:128, 1954.
35. Trantas, M.   Kératite ponctuée lepréuse, Arch. opht., 32:193, 1912.
36. Tsutsui, J.   Tetanus infection of the cornea, Am. J. Ophth., 43:772, 1957.
37. Vaughan, D. G., Jr.   Corneal ulcers, Surv. Ophth., 3:203, 1958.
38. Weeks, J. E.   Tuberculosis of the eye, Am. J. Ophth., 9:243, 1926.
39. Weeks, J. E.   The bacillus of acute conjunctival catarrh, or "pink eye," Arch. Ophth., 15:441, 1886.
40. Weiss, C., Shevky, M. C., and Perry, I. H.   Experimental investigation of the pathogenicity of diphtheroids isolated from the human conjunctiva, Arch. Ophth., 40:23, 1948.
41. Wilson, G. S., and Miles, A. A.   Topley and Wilson's Principles of Bacteriology and Immunity, 4th ed., Baltimore, The Williams & Wilkins Co., 1955.

GRAM-NEGATIVE GROUP

NEISSERIA

The members of this genus are gram-negative cocci, typically intracellular and arranged in pairs. Except in the case of the gonococcus, they are normal inhabitants of the nasopharynx in man, healthy or ill.

Only neisseria of medical interest will be discussed:

> *Neisseria gonorrhoeae*
> *Neisseria meningitidis*
> *Neisseria catarrhalis*

Neisseria gonorrhoeae

The gonococcus was first described by Neisser in 1879, when he isolated the organism from purulent urethritis and vaginitis. Gonorrhea is the most prevalent of the venereal diseases. The sensitivity of the gonococcus to sulfonamides and penicillin has greatly decreased the incidence of acute infection. However, resistant strains are no longer rare. More important is the fact that diseases may become chronic in persons who seem to have been cured and where laboratory tests reveal no organisms.

Extragenital gonococcal infection may occur: cystitis, stomatitis, and more often, conjunctivitis in the newborn (ophthalmia neonatorum).

The infection may invade the blood; septicemia, arthritis, and endocarditis are among the sequelae.

Morphology. Smears reveal *N. gonorrhoeae* to be mainly a typical kidney-shaped diplococcus. Isolated cocci and those from cultures are round, resembling staphylococci. While *N. gonorrhoeae* may be found extracellularly, usually in a chronic process, intracellular occurrence within leukocytes is more characteristic, being important for diagnosis (Plate XIII, 3A). The organism stains readily with methylene blue alone. Difficulties arise with the gram stain because gonococci are not always readily decolorized, or the involution forms found in culture are often swollen and take the stain poorly. The organisms retaining stain may be mistaken for staphylococci. To obtain a good stain, one must prepare as thin and uniform a film as possible. This will allow a microscopic diagnosis of the smear secretion.

Culture. The gonococci require enriched media. While many different media are used, growth may be obtained with the simplest of them, such as chocolate or blood agar, particularly in an atmosphere containing 10 per cent CO_2. The CO_2 atmosphere can be produced with a candle jar. Since the gonococci require moisture, a piece of moist blotting paper should be placed on the bottom of the jar along with the inoculated plate. The gonococci are easily autolyzed and die rapidly, hence incubation should not be longer than 48 hours. They grow best at a slightly lower than normal incubation temperature, 35 to 36°C. The material should be swabbed into a broth and brought to the laboratory immediately, then inoculated, as gonococci die rapidly at room temperature.

On chocolate agar, colonies are unpigmented, glistening, large, mucoid, and semitranslucent. They have irregular edges, do not produce hemolysis, and are odorless (Plate XIII, 6).

Members of the *Neisseria* genus produce oxidase and autolytic enzymes. Therefore, the oxidase test is common to all neisseria. The test is used to identify colonies of the *Neisseria* genus and to distinguish them in mixed, overcrowded plates. For the test, the dye solution (1 per cent of dimethyl or tetramethyl para-phenylenediamine) must be dropped on the suspicious area. The oxidase-positive colonies turn from pink to red to black. When the color is black, the organism is dead (Plate XIV, 5). Some of the gram-negative bacilli show a positive oxidase test, but their color is gray instead of black.

For differential diagnosis of the species, the fermentation test is necessary. The gonococcus ferments dextrose but does not ferment maltose or sucrose (Plate XIII, 5).

Antigenic Structure. It is difficult to establish definite serologic types, since the majority of strains are antigenically related. There are, however, two main antigenic types: Type I, usually involved in an acute process, and Type II, in chronic processes. Between these two there are a number of intermediate types containing one or more common antigens.

Gonococcal polysaccharides and nucleoproteins are not specific and are similar to those of the meningococcus. Permanent immunity does not develop.

Pathogenicity and Virulence. The gonococcus is very restricted as to its human portal of entry; it attacks mainly the mucous membranes of the genitourinary tract and the conjunctiva. The disease process is acutely purulent; it is usually local. Blood invasion occurs rarely, and arthritis (very painful), endocarditis, or other conditions may develop, all probably of toxic origin.

The gonococcus produces an endotoxin which can be extracted from the organisms. The endotoxin may be liberated from the culture by autolysis of the bacteria.

The resistance of the gonococcus is very low; it is easily destroyed by drying and by heat, even as low as 30°C, within five minutes.

Findings in the Eye. The gonococcus may cause a violent acute purulent conjunctivitis which may be complicated by ulceration of the cornea, with resultant scarring and blindness. Two types are clinically distinguished: gonococcal conjunctivitis of the newborn (ophthalmia neonatorum) and gonococcal conjunctivitis of the adult.

GONOCOCCAL CONJUNCTIVITIS IN THE NEWBORN (OPHTHALMIA NEONATORUM). While the condition is not common where the law requires prophylaxis, it may still develop.[5] It results from gonorrheal urethritis of the mother. The infant's eyes are infected during the passage through the birth canal; extremely rarely does ocular infection occur in utero. The incubation period of ophthalmia neonatorum is one to three days, and usually involvement is bilateral. At onset there is a sanious discharge which then becomes purulent (Plate XIII, 2) and so copious that it may flow down the cheek. Sometimes pseudomembranes may develop. The markedly swollen lids are difficult to open, and pus accumulates in the conjunctival sac. Glasses should be worn before opening the child's lids, or pus may spray into the observer's eyes and cause a severe ocular infection. In spite of the copious purulent discharge, the conjunctival tissue may at first be only slightly involved. Later, it becomes very red and rough. On this basis, gonococcal conjunctivitis is differentiated from the other bacterial conjunctivitides in the newborn. For instance, in staphylococcal infections, the conjunctiva is only slightly involved.

Gonococcal ophthalmia, particularly in severe or untreated cases, is commonly complicated by a severe purulent type of keratitis. It is associated with the period of discharge and marked edema of the lids. The pressure by the swollen lids decreases the blood supply, and toxic pus macerates the corneal epithelium, thus creating a portal of entry. The keratitis begins as a yellowish infiltrate which progresses and ulcerates very rapidly, with resulting perforation and panophthalmitis.

The disease is highly contagious, and isolation of the child is mandatory.

In children's hospital wards, schools, or orphanages, epidemics of vulvovaginitis or infantile purulent conjunctivitis may occur. The conjunctivitis is caused by staphylococci, streptococci, or other bacteria, but the gonococcus is the prime offender . It usually occurs in girls aged 2 to 10, transmitted by direct sexual contact or deviation. In our laboratory, the gonococcus was isolated from a sporadic case of infantile purulent conjunctivitis in a 5 year old girl. The contact was not established (Plate XIII, 1). Laboratory examination is essential for differential diagnosis.

GONOCOCCAL CONJUNCTIVITIS IN THE ADULT. This condition is usually unilateral and results from self-transmission of the organism from the urethral tract. Therefore, it occurs mainly in males, and the right eye is most frequently involved. The clinical picture while similar to ophthalmia neonatorum has certain differences: the purulent discharge is not as copious; the conjunctival tissue tends to be more involved and becomes more papillary and rougher than in children. The most important characteristic is that the cornea is almost constantly involved; until the antibiotic era, many eyes were lost. As in children, the possible consequences are perforation of the cornea, endophthalmitis, and panophthalmitis.

Iritis, iridocyclitis with hypopyon (without involvement of the cornea), or lid abscess may develop.

Even now, the prognosis in adults must be guarded.

Prophylaxis. The classical prophylaxis by Credé, proposed in 1880, consisted of instillation of 1 drop of 1 per cent silver nitrate solution into each eye of the newborn. Its requirement by law in most parts of the world brought a great advance in the prevention of gonococcal conjunctivitis. The method has recently been re-evaluated in view of irritation by the silver nitrate, and instead, prophylaxis by antibiotics has been advocated.[27] However, a new problem arose: sensitivity of the host to antibiotics, especially penicillin. As a result some go as far as to omit any prophylaxis, since antibiotic action is specific for gonococcal infection. However, an increase of gonococcal conjunctivitis in the newborn was reported. Therefore, prophylaxis still is the accepted procedure, although not necessarily by Credé's method. If silver nitrate is used, the lid margin first must be thoroughly cleansed with dry cotton, then the silver nitrate instilled. It is important that this be in contact with the entire conjunctiva.

In adults, the normal eye should be protected by Buller's or some other shield.

Diagnosis. The typical clinical picture and study of a properly prepared smear may be satisfactory for diagnosis. The organisms are more easily seen in the beginning period of purulent discharge. For early diagnosis of gonococcal conjunctivitis, particularly in adults, scraping is preferable to smear. It shows gonococci on the epithelial cells prior to finding them in the secretion (Plate XIII, 4). A culture is necessary in a case of negative smear and in order to confirm the diagnosis. Gonococci may remain in the conjunctiva after the clinical symptoms disappear.

Neisseria meningitidis
(Meningococcus)

The meningococcus is of great importance in medicine as it causes epidemics of cerebrospinal meningitis which can often be fatal. Man is the only known natural host of pathogenic meningococci. These intracellular diplococci have a morphology similar to the gonococcus (Plate XIV, 2, 3). Culture requirements and characteristics are also similar except that the meningococcus ferments glucose and maltose but not sucrose (Plate XIV, 4). (For details, see page 44.

The meningococci have been separated into four major groups, A, B, C, and D, corresponding to the old classification of Types I, II, III, and IV. Group D or Type IV is rarely found in the United States. Groups A and C have capsules which react with specific antisera and result in Quellung similar to that found in the pneumococcus. Each type may be identified through agglutination tests with specific sera.

Pathogenicity and Virulence.   The nucleoproteins of N. *meningitidis* are regarded as endotoxins, but they are not specific. Toxicity is probably due to some constituents of the nucleoproteins. No immunity develops.

Clinical Features.   The meningococcus is a specific cause of purulent epidemic cerebrospinal meningitis, especially in children. Epidemics have a tendency to cyclic occurrence at about 8 to 12 year intervals. The most severe cases occur in adults, especially soldiers. A severe outbreak in the United States was recorded at the beginning of World War II (1940-1943).

If the organisms reach the blood stream meningococcemia develops, which is usually characterized by purpuric spots, due to thrombosis of the capillaries. Meningococci may be cultured from these spots, especially in an early stage. Meningococcemia may become chronic.

The source of infection is usually a healthy carrier or a person who has recovered from the disease. The nasopharynx is the major portal and harbor of infection; in persons exposed, it must be examined and treated during an epidemic.

Findings in the Eye.   Meningococcal ocular infections are increasingly discussed in the literature. In 1944 and 1946, a considerable number of cases were reported.[29, 37, 41, 46] Acute conjunctivitis is the most common manifestation. This is purulent, sometimes resembling gonococcal conjunctivitis, and occasionally occurs in the newborn. The conjunctivitis may be complicated by various types of keratitis. Among them are mild ulceration and multiple stromal infiltration; in a case reported by Allen the latter showed peripheral diffuse circular bands. More rarely endophthalmitis may develop. Free meningococci have been reported in a case of keratomalacia. In our laboratory, meningococci were isolated from pus of opened meibomitis. Another patient, a boy of 12, developed mild purulent meningococcal conjunctivitis and a few stromal infiltrates of the cornea. An additional case of keratitis is illustrated in Plate XIV, 1. The laboratory investigation of material from the inflamed meibomian gland seemed reasonable. It is probable that the glands can harbor meningococci.

The ocular condition may occur independently or as a complication of the meningitis.[26] Papillitis is most frequently found; among the other complications, retinitis, subconjunctival hemorrhages, and endophthalmitis may occur.

On the other hand, the infection from the eye can invade the blood, causing meningococcemia and meningitis.

Fortunately, meningococcal infection has usually been successfully treated with sulfonamides and penicillin.

It must be stressed that meningococcal ocular infection is much more frequent than might be realized. Meningococci can also be found in normal flora, being a potential source of infection. Therefore, complete study of the culture and serologic differentiation of the *Neisseria* genus is important.

Treatment. Penicillin in high doses is usually effective treatment. Even in those cases in which conjunctivitis is the only manifestation of meningococcal infection, local therapy plus intensive systemic treatment by sulfadiazine or penicillin should be employed to prevent meningitis. During epidemics, it is advisable to investigate normal flora of the conjunctiva of persons exposed, and if meningococci are found, the introduction of sulfonamides, especially of sulfadiazine ointment, may be useful for prophylaxis.

Neisseria catarrhalis

Neisseria catarrhalis is a constant inhabitant of the respiratory tract. While this member of the *Neisseria* genus is generally considered saprophytic, it can at times be weakly pathogenic. *N. catarrhalis* may be confused with *N. meningitidis*, since both are inhabitants of the pharynx; differential diagnosis is of great importance.

Morphologically in the smear secretion it is indistinguishable from gonococci and meningococci. It is coffee bean-shaped and intracellular (Plate XV, 1). Nonetheless, these cocci may be larger than other neisseria and may stain more intensely.

Cultural differentiation is most significant. *N. catarrhalis,* unlike other neisseria, grows abundantly and freely on ordinary media. On plain agar the colonies are round, gray, and glistening, but after 24 hours of incubation they become opaque and slightly brown in the center (Plate XV, 5). Their tendency to autoagglutinate makes it very difficult and practically impossible to achieve a uniform suspension.

Biochemically, *N. catarrhalis* does not produce acid or gas from any of the sugars. Fermentation tests with maltose, glucose, and sucrose are negative (Plate XV, 4). *N. catarrhalis* is more resistant to physical agents than are gonococci and meningococci.

Findings in the Eye.   Although principally nonpathogenic, *N. catarrhalis* may become a pathogen in certain eye conditions. It is occasionally found in mild and even severe cases of conjunctivitis and in postoperative conjunctivitis. The organism is found most frequently in cases of inflammation of the meibomian glands.

An extremely rare case of endophthalmitis due to *N. catarrhalis* has been reported.[20]

Summary

For differentiation of neisseria, fermentation tests are most important:

	MALTOSE	GLUCOSE	SUCROSE
Neisseria gonorrhoeae	−	+	−
Neisseria meningitidis	+	+	−
Neisseria catarrhalis	−	−	−

N. catarrhalis is distinguished by the fact that it grows on ordinary media.

MORAXELLA GENUS

Moraxella lacunata
(Morax-Axenfeld Diplobacillus)

The Morax-Axenfeld diplobacillus, while of little interest in other medical fields, has particular importance for the ophthalmologist. This organism is responsible for ocular diseases alone, and therefore general bacteriologists have given it little attention.

The organism was described by Morax in 1896 and independently by Axenfeld in 1897. While Morax-Axenfeld diplobacillus is its most common name, others such as *Bacillus lacunata, Hemophilus lacunata* and *Hemophilus duplex* have been used. This multiple nomenclature would indicate confusion in classification of the organism. While sometimes considered in the group of miscellaneous organisms, it is now regarded as in the *Moraxella* genus, closely related to *Haemophilus. Moraxella lacunata* (Morax-Axenfeld diplobacillus) and *Moraxella liquefaciens* (diplobacillus of Petit) are members of the genus *Moraxella*.

Morphology.   This is the largest gram-negative bacillus causing ocular diseases. In the secretion the bacilli are short, but stout, with intensively staining (polar stain) rectangular or round ends. While usually arranged in pairs—hence diplobacilli—the organisms may at times appear in short chains, and capsules may be present (Plate XVI, 3B). The secretion is characteristically mucoid, with fibrin threads, and it is not purulent. Numerous organisms are usually found, either free or within epithelial cells, even in the mild, almost asymptomatic process. *M. lacunata* may proliferate on the surface of desquamated epithelium. This organism has a typical morphology in secretion, and thus diagnosis is possible from a study of the smear alone. The morphology changes quickly in the culture (Plate XVI, 3A). Only during the first day can one find typical diplobacillary or streptobacillary forms; later, one may find forms varying from very long thin filaments to short coccobacilli. The variations in this respect are so marked that in our laboratory, Horwich and Fedukowicz believe they have demonstrated a linkage to the micrococcus recently described by Mitsui and associates. Sometimes the cells of *M. lacunata* become club-shaped, thus resembling corynebacteria. In the same slide gram-negative and gram-positive diplobacilli may simultaneously be found. The long diplobacilli usually stain pale pink, whereas the short stout coccobacilli may be gram-positive.

The organisms are nonmotile, nonsporing aerobes.

Culture. *M. lacunata* requires enriched media. Generally it grows on any medium containing animal serum. Löffler's serum medium is certainly the most practical for the ophthalmologist. Pits are formed on this medium, demonstrating the degree of liquefaction, an important characteristic for identification (Plate XVI, 4). While no actual colonies are visible on the medium, the surface is covered by circumscribed pits of liquefaction, hence the term *lacunata*. On blood agar, the colonies develop slowly. They are grayish, semitransparent, mucoid, usually nonhemolytic, and odorless (Plate XVI, 5). There is no growth on chocolate agar, and there is no fermentation of sugars. It is important that any medium used have an alkaline reaction. *M. lacunata* grows in symbiosis with *Corynebacterium xerosis,* an organism that does not produce any acid. On the other hand, the organism usually does not grow in the presence of the acid-producing *Staphylococcus aureus.* In direct smear, *S. aureus* is rarely found when *M. lacunata* is present.

Resistance. According to the literature, these diplobacilli usually die after about 10 days of subcultivation. In our laboratory, we have been able to keep cultures alive for almost three weeks by transferring them every other day. Dried organisms may remain alive four days or longer. The diplobacillus can be killed in one to five minutes by moist heat at 58°C.

Pathogenicity. As far as is known, *M. lacunata* is pathogenic only for the eye, causing the typical clinical picture of angular blepharoconjunctivitis or hypopyon keratitis. It is suggested that these diplobacilli produce the enzyme protease, which can be inhibited by tears (believed to contain antiprotease). Hence it is possible that bacilli try to escape to the angulus from the conjunctiva which is bathed in tears. Angular blepharoconjunctivitis then develops.

This organism has been regarded as nonpathogenic for animals; however, this view is no longer correct. White mice may die within 24 hours after intraperitoneal injection of a suspension of the culture (Oeding).[38] However, animal passage is negative. We have observed that intracorneal inoculation of strains isolated from hypopyon keratitis produces a deep hypopyon keratitis in rabbits.

Findings in the Eye.   Chronic angular blepharoconjunctivitis is an al-most pathognomonic indication for *M. lacunata* infection. While rare in most of the United States, the disease is not uncommon in Arizona and New Mexico. Epidemics have occurred, but they have not been severe. In gen-eral the condition is endemic, particularly in institutions (personal observa-tions in institutions for the retarded). The disease predominantly affects adults, during hot dusty seasons or in hot climates; however, cases have been reported in the newborn.

Blepharoconjunctivitis is a chronic process which may last for years, characterized by redness, particularly of the outer anguli (Plate XVI, 1). Numerous diplobacilli can be isolated from this site, even in very mild con-ditions. These mild cases may easily be overlooked and, if untreated, may cause postoperative infections.

M. lacunata very rarely causes a severe acute conjunctivitis similar to blennorrhea.

The cornea may show a marginal type of ulceration similar to any other ulcer associated with bacterial conjunctivitis.

A central hypopyon keratitis, typically in abscess form, may occur pri-marily (without preceding blepharoconjunctivitis), particularly in alcoholic and debilitated persons (Plate XVI, 2). A history of preceding ocular trauma is commonly elicited. Hypopyon keratitis due to the Morax-Axenfeld diplo-bacillus is the predominant type found at Bellevue Hospital, in contrast to the high incidence of pneumococcal keratitis reported elsewhere (Feduko-wicz and Horwich).[16] The process spreads deeply, possibly to avoid contact with tears, and painlessly, with development of an intracorneal abscess. Sometimes two zones of infiltration are seen: a central one separated by a clear zone from a peripheral one. A posterior abscess may occur.

At onset, the surface of the cornea over the abscess may appear intact. Later, necrosis and ulceration develop. Scraping the cornea is of value only after the cornea breaks down. First the necrotic mass is cleaned away, then the ulcer base must be scraped, since it is here that the bacilli reside (not in the margin, as in the case of pneumococcal ulcer). Perforation of the cornea or secondary glaucoma may often result.

Treatment.   Zinc salts appear to have an almost specific action upon diplobacillary infections. In cases of blepharoconjunctivitis a 0.25 per cent to 0.5 per cent solution of zinc sulfate, three times a day, is recommended. To treat keratitis, zinc sulfate in high concentrations is used, but with extreme caution and only if the cornea has not been too thinned by the process. Successful treatment of corneal ulcer by cauterization with a zinc sulfate solution as concentrated as 20 per cent is recorded (Duke-Elder). However, cauterization with 5 or 10 per cent solution of zinc sulfate is effective in the early stages of the keratitis. In this technic, the following steps should be followed: the eye must be thoroughly anesthetized topically, since cauterization is a painful procedure. For cauterization, a thin applicator

Plates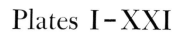

PLATE I

1. Chronic ulcerative blepharitis due to staphylococci. Ulcers at roots of lashes are covered by dry crusts. The process may last for years. Avoid overtreatment. Antibiotics to be chosen according to sensitivity test. Remove crusts before taking specimen; use wet saline swab. Smear and culture are necessary.

2. Hordeolum internum (meibomitis) due to staphylococci. This condition is often associated with blepharitis; it may be multiple and recurrent. Characterized by pain and localized swelling. A yellow spot is usually seen through the conjunctiva. Preauricular glands are often enlarged.

3. Catarrhal marginal ulcer of cornea, the usual consequence of staphylococcal blepharoconjunctivitis. Single or several superficial infiltrates are separated from the limbus by a clear zone. Infiltrates easily ulcerate. No bacteria are found. The condition is regarded as allergic or toxic.

4. Acute catarrhal conjunctivitis due to staphylococci. Palpebral conjunctiva, especially of lower lid, is involved. Discharge is purulent. Acute process often becomes chronic, with associated blepharitis.

5. Varied morphology of staphylococci.

A. Staphylococci from panophthalmitis (scraping, Giemsa stain). Unusual, intracellular, kidney-shaped diplococci predominate (can be confused with gonococci). Culture and gram stain confirm diagnosis. Note neutrophils.

B. Staphylococci from blepharoconjunctivitis (smear, gram stain). May be diagnosed in direct smear by round shape, regular size, and clusterlike arrangement. Culture is needed for pathogenicity and sensitivity tests, and to confirm diagnosis.

6. Cultures of *Staphylococcus aureus, albus,* and *citreus* (see page 13). Colonies circular, discrete, elevated, opaque, and glistening. Strains are distinguished by pigments.

A. *Staphylococcus citreus* (lemon-yellow). This has a drier appearance than the others. Nonpathogenic.

B. *Staphylococcus aureus* (golden yellow). Usually pathogenic

C. *Staphylococcus albus* (white). Mainly nonpathogenic.

PLATE I 49

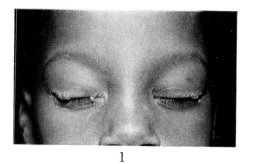

1

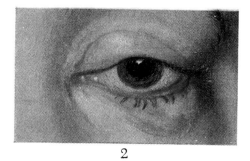

2

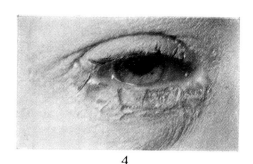

3

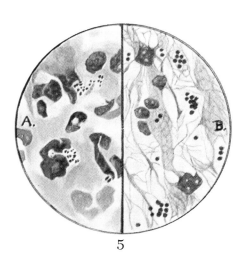

4

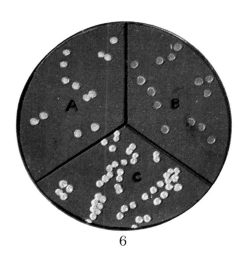

5

6

PLATE II

1. Chronic blepharitis. This process is of long duration. Observe the thickening of lid margins (tylosis ciliaris); also note that only a few atrophic cilia remain (madarosis).

2. Sebaceous cyst (atheroma). Considered to be a retention cyst, this may grow to considerable size. The usual location is the inner canthus, which may cause confusion with dacryocystitis. Staphylococci are isolated.

3. Coagulase test. A slide with two drops of bacterial emulsion. The dark area on each shows where human plasma has been added. White spots indicate coagulation (see page 14).
   A. Negative.
   B. Positive.

4. Staphylococcus in original culture on blood agar. Isolated from blepharitis. The coagulase test was positive, showing pathogenicity of this *albus* strain.

5. Disk sensitivity test. This shows a resistant strain of staphylococcus, obviously sensitive to Albamycin and slightly to Chloromycetin.

6. Varied morphology of staphylococci (smear from culture).
   A. From panophthalmitis. Among typical round cocci are a few kidney-shaped staphylococci.
   B. From blepharitis. Illustrates typical morphology: round shape, regularity of size and staining, and clusterlike arrangement.

PLATE II 51

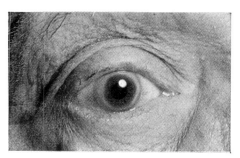

1

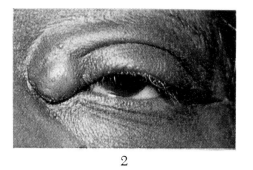

2

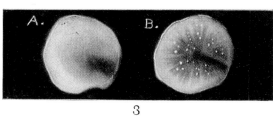

3

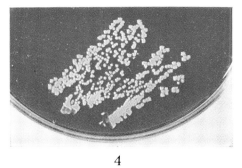

4

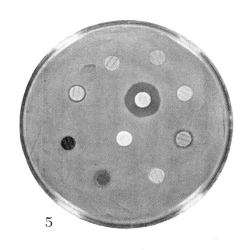

5

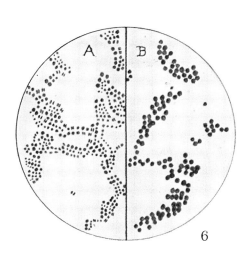

6

PLATE III

1. Pneumococcal acute mucopurulent conjunctivitis. Most frequent type of acute bacterial conjunctivitis. Moderate severity; mild mucopurulent exudation. Pronounced redness of bulbar conjunctiva; petechiae (frequent on upper bulbar conjunctiva; rarely found on lower). Note follicles in lower fornix. Marginal or punctate keratitis may occur.

2. Pneumococcal hypopyon ulcer (serpiginous type). Beginning stage of purulent, very destructive keratitis. This may result in perforation and panophthalmitis. Infection is usually secondary to corneal abrasion. The condition is often associated with chronic dacryocystitis. Hypopyon is sterile and indicates acute iritis. The progressive margin is undermined. Take specimen from this pocket, by loop.

3. Granulomatous masses following acute suppurative dacryocystitis.

4. Acute suppurative dacryocystitis. Pus discharged from opening, typically below lacrimal sac. The pneumococcus is the most common pathogen.

5. Exudate (original smear) from acute pneumococcal conjunctivitis, illustrating encapsulated lancet-shaped diplococci. Eosinophilic cell may indicate an allergic reaction to infection.

6. Smear from hypopyon ulcer. Typical lancet-shaped pneumococci permit diagnosis by direct smear. Occasional partially lysed cells are present.

PLATE III 53

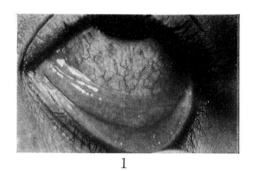

1

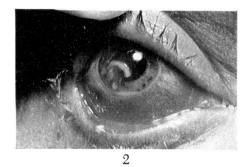

2

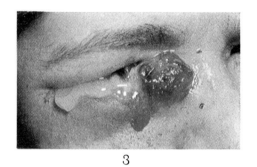

3

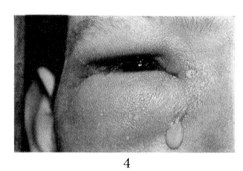

4

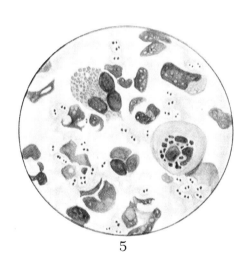

5

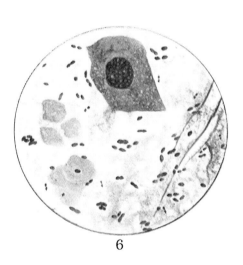

6

PLATE IV

1. Capsule stain (Hiss copper sulfate method). Heavy, unstained capsule seen against violet background.

2. Pneumococci from blood agar culture. Morphology differs from that in the original smear; here, the pneumococci are irregular in size and with less marked diplo arrangement. Note the distinct capsule, which differentiates the pneumococcus from *Streptococcus mitis* (alpha).

3. Optochin sensitivity test. Place the optochin disk on a blood agar culture of pneumococci. Unlike alpha streptococci, it shows a zone of inhibition indicating sensitivity to optochin.

    A. Pneumococcus.

    B. Alpha streptococci.

4. Culture of pneumococci on blood agar. Tiny, glistening colonies, surrounded by a green zone of incomplete alpha hemolysis (indistinguishable from *Streptococcus mitis*).

5. Bile solubility test to differentiate streptococcus from the pneumococcus. Tube on left, with opaque appearance, demonstrates insolubility of *Streptococcus mitis*. Clear, transparent contents of tube at right indicate solubility of *Diplococcus pneumoniae*.

PLATE IV   55

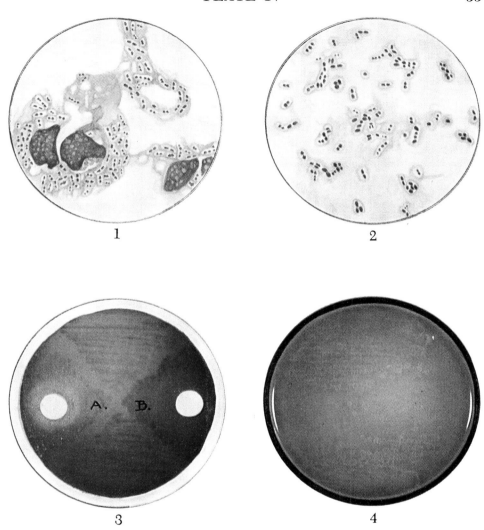

1

2

3

4

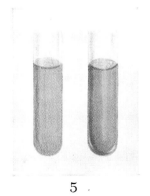

5

PLATE V

1. *Streptococcus mitis* (alpha) endophthalmitis. Yellow exudate in pupillary area and synechia posterior.

2. Central hypopyon ulcer. This may be more severe than pneumococcal ulcer (see Plate III, 2).

3. Posterior abscess due to *Streptococcus pyogenes*. This condition is rare, found in extremely virulent infection. Exudate in posterior layers of cornea. Descemet's membrane bulges and may rupture into anterior chamber.

4. Morphologic characteristics of *Streptococcus mitis*.

    A. Original exudate from hypopyon ulcer (gram stain). Elongated cocci in diplo or short chain arrangement. No capsule.

    B. Smear from Brewer's culture. In fluid medium, long chains develop.

5. Culture of *Streptococcus mitis* on blood agar is similar to pneumococcal culture; the colonies are small, flat, and surrounded by a green zone of incomplete alpha hemolysis.

PLATE V   57

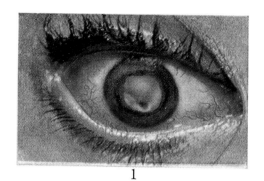

1

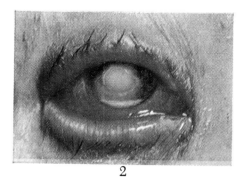

2

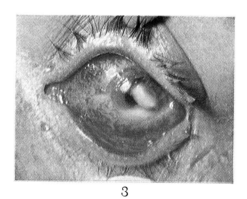

3

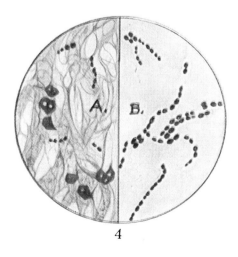

4

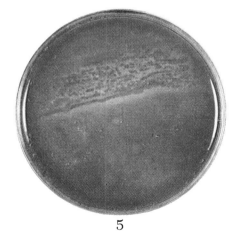

5

PLATE VI

1. True membranous conjunctivitis due to *Streptococcus pyogenes* (beta). Co-agulative fibrinous exudate, penetrating interepithelial spaces and subepithelial tissue, forms a heavy membrane. Unlike *Corynebacterium diphtheriae*, the membrane may develop on bulbar conjunctiva also.

2. *Streptococcus pyogenes* culture on blood agar. Important characteristics: small, pointed, opaque colonies surrounded by a big zone (2 to 5 mm or extended area) of complete beta hemolysis.

3. *Streptococcus pyogenes* in smears from culture (gram stain). Diplo or short chain arrangements found in cultures on solid medium (blood agar). The same streptococci show long chains in fluid medium (Brewer).

4. Cellulitis of the upper lid due to *Streptococcus pyogenes*. A history of injury is usual. Process in late stage shows extensive sloughing due to necrosis. The cornea is not involved. The preauricular node is not enlarged. Consequences may be heavy scarring, ectropion, or lagophthalmos.

5. Panophthalmitis due to *Streptococcus pyogenes*. All structures of the eye show suppurative inflammation. Tremendous chemosis, swelling, and redness of lids. Infiltration of Tenon's capsule causes exophthalmos.

PLATE VI

59

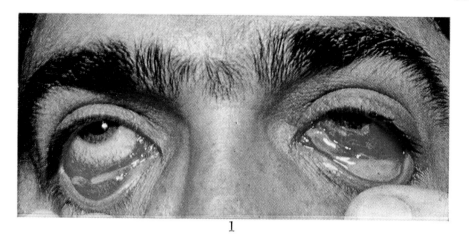

1

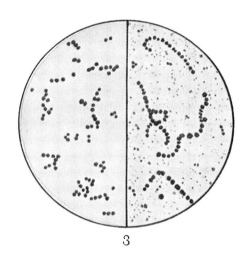

2

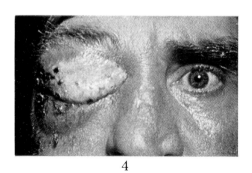

3

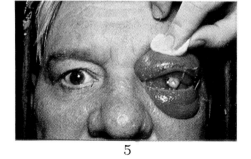

4

5

PLATE VII

1. *Corynebacterium xerosis* in scraping (Giemsa stain). C. xerosis is the most frequent and most confusing organism found in the eye. Often gives diplococcal appearance (when metachromatic granules present at poles). Important characteristics: uninterrupted wall, irregular size and shape, no capsule, and found on degenerated "keratinized" epithelium.

2. *C. xerosis* in smears from culture on blood agar (showing variety of morphology).

    A. From young culture: bacilli smaller and more regular; typically arranged in clumps and V formations.

    B. From old culture: bacilli have confusing morphology. Metachromatic granules give appearance of streptococci or diplococci. Uninterrupted body wall and irregularities of size and shape (club-shaped bodies), V, L, and palisade arrangement are important clues.

3. Bitot's spot. Foamy white, dry, lusterless spot localized in temporal or nasal interpalpebral zone of bulbar conjunctiva. Condition often associated with night blindness. Scraping shows "keratinized" epithelium containing numerous *C. xerosis* bacilli.

4. Keratomalacia. Usually occurs in children. The condition causes complete destruction of the cornea, associated with debility and malnutrition. *C. xerosis* bacilli are invariably present in large numbers.

5. *C. xerosis* culture on blood agar.

    A. Dustlike, opaque colonies with dry appearance. Growth is slow (two to seven days).

    B. Culture with unusually dry, crusted appearance. *C. xerosis* alone was identified. Isolated from a Puerto Rican patient with an old trachoma.

6. Metachromatic granules (Neisser stain). Important indication for differential diagnosis: limited number of dark metachromatic granules distributed throughout the body of *C. xerosis*.

PLATE VII 61

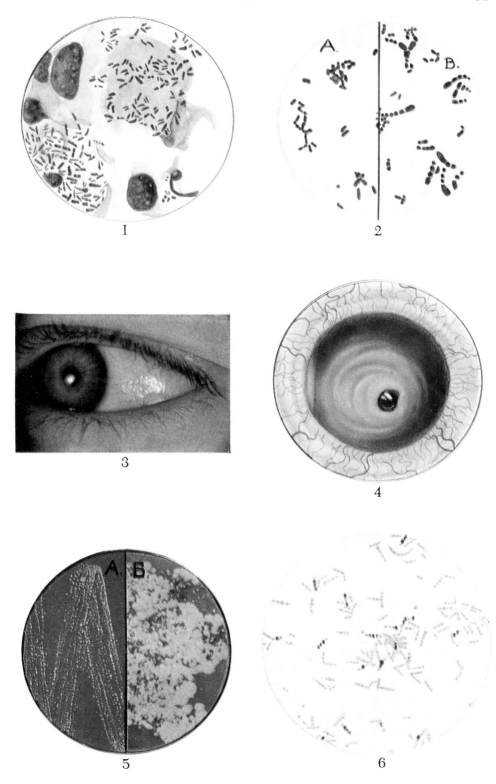

PLATE VIII

1. Diphtheritic membranous conjunctivitis. Membrane develops on tarsal conjunctiva. It is composed of yellowish gray, coagulated necrotic material embedded in exuded fibrin. Interepithelial spaces and subepithelial tissue are penetrated. When membrane is removed, bleeding occurs. Conjunctivitis may be complicated by severe purulent keratitis.

2. Diphtheritic mucopurulent conjunctivitis. Indistinguishable from other bacterial conjunctivitides. Characterized by mucopurulent discharge without true membrane.

3. Metachromatic granules of *C. diphtheriae* (Neisser stain). Granules are moderate in number and located at poles, giving a drumstick appearance. Cultures and virulence test are needed for diagnosis.

4. *Corynebacterium diphtheriae* cultures.

   A. Tellurite medium. Intracellular reduction of tellurite causes a gunmetal color of the colonies. Center is darker than the periphery (see page 25).

   B. Blood agar. Colonies are gray and opaque. Unlike staphylococcal colonies, they are dull.

5. *C. diphtheriae* on Löffler's serum. Colonies are small, creamy, granular, and moist.

PLATE VIII 63

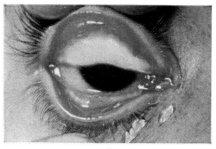

1

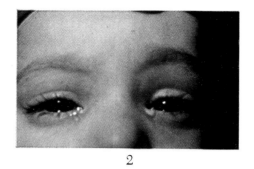

2

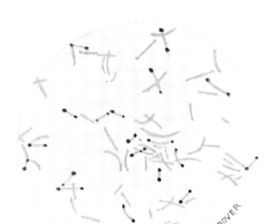

3

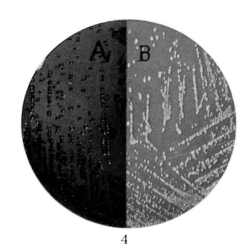

4

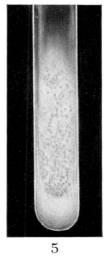

5

PLATE IX

1. *Corynebacterium diphtheriae* and *Corynebacterium xerosis* in smears from culture (Neisser stain).

A. *C. diphtheriae*. Metachromatic granules are more numerous than in *C. xerosis* and typically located at poles, giving a drumstick appearance.

B. *C. xerosis*. Metachromatic granules seen in small numbers. Unlike *C. diphtheriae*, these are located throughout the entire organism.

2. In vitro test for virulence. Three streaks show growth of three different strains of corynebacteria. Radiating lines (exaggerated by retouching) seen at streak B indicate that this is the only virulent strain of the three (see page 27).

3. *C. diphtheriae* and *C. xerosis* cultures.

On blood agar:

A. *C. diphtheriae* colonies are larger than *C. xerosis*.

B. *C. xerosis* colonies are smaller and drier than *C. diphtheriae*.

On Löffler's serum:

C. *C. diphtheriae* colonies are larger (also faster growing than on blood agar; important for early diagnosis).

D. *C. xerosis* is smaller and drier than *C. diphtheriae* (growth slower).

4. Fermentation reactions of *C. diphtheriae*.

Glucose: positive (yellow).

Sucrose: negative (red).

5. Fermentation reaction of *C. xerosis*.

Glucose: positive (yellow).

The reaction with sucrose is also positive.

PLATE IX

65

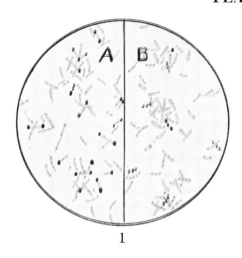

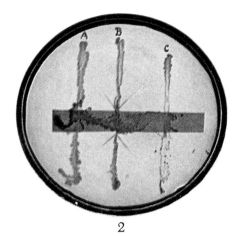

1

2

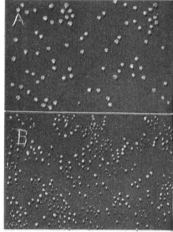

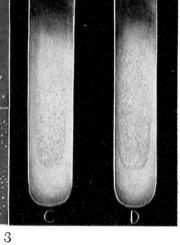

3

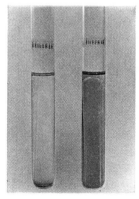

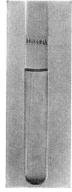

4

5

PLATE X

1. Primary tuberculosis of conjunctiva. Tarsal conjunctiva, which is mainly involved, is much thickened. Conjunctivitis is the papillary type. On top of the papillae, an ulcer often develops, as shown. The condition is associated with oculoglandular Parinaud's syndrome.

2. Deep interstitial keratitis. The keratitis is often in the upper outer quadrant. Vessels penetrate the lesion deeply, in characteristic distribution (unbranched, disappearing at limbus).

3. Unusual, acute, exudative type of ocular tuberculosis. Marked destruction of globe by coalescent necrosis, with resultant cavities. Original smear showed numerous tubercle bacilli. Association with hypersensitivity is assumed.

4. Original smear (Ziehl-Neelsen stain). Acid-fast tubercle bacilli, having granular appearance, arranged predominantly in V forms and resembling corynebacteria.

5. Culture of tubercle bacilli on Löwenstein-Jensen medium (malachite prevents contamination and gives a beautiful green color). Colonies are creamy, dull, rough, and granular. Growth requires at least two months.

PLATE X   67

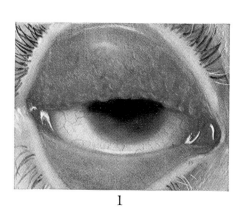

1

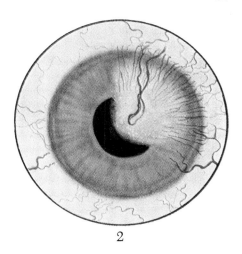

2

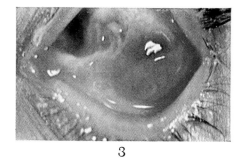

3

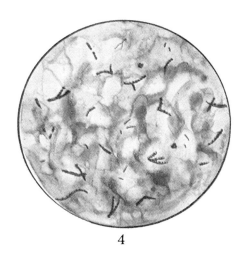

4

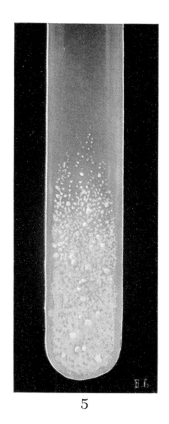

5

PLATE XI

1. Phlyctenular conjunctivitis. Several small grayish white limbal nodules. Phlyctenules tend to ulcerate (see page 33).

2. Fascicular keratitis. Note phlyctenule migrating across the cornea, with accompanying vascular tail. (It may extend from limbus to limbus.) The end stage will be a permanent, superficial ribbonlike opacity crossing the cornea.

3. Perforating pustular phlyctenule. Phlyctenules may become acute, purulent, and penetrating. Prolapse of the iris is shown. Perforation then results in adherent leukoma or anterior staphyloma.

4. Eczematous (scrofulous, phlyctenular) pannus. This pannus may involve any or all of the peripheral cornea (trachomatous pannus involves the upper cornea). Superficial vessels beneath the epithelium show arborescent branching.

PLATE XI 69

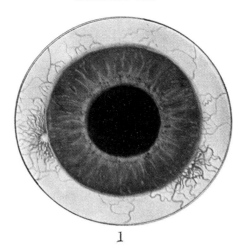

1

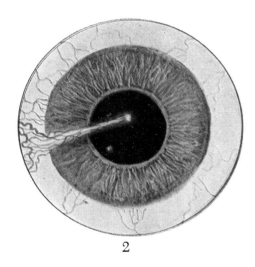

2

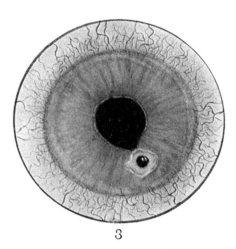

3

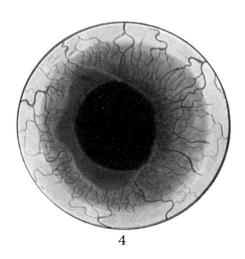

4

PLATE XII

1. Leprotic keratitis. Slit lamp view; small, white opacities and scattered, chalky, minute grains seen in all layers. Note the nodules on the thickened nerves. Hansen's bacilli were found in the corneal scraping. (From patient shown at right.)

2. Nodular leprosy (lepra tuberosa; lepromatous leprosy). Nodules, single or grouped, are typically distributed on the face, mainly on the cheeks, lips, and nose.

3. Multiple, irregular, quiet retinal lesions at the periphery of the fundus. (Same patient as in 2, above.) The lesions are probably of leprotic origin.

4. Hansen's bacilli in scraping. (From keratitis in 1, above.) Acid-fast bacilli vary in size and shape. They may be straight, curved, arranged in palisade and V formation, or granular globules. Scraping is sufficient for diagnosis; Hansen's bacilli have never been cultivated.

5. Corneal leproma. A large, nodular conglomeration (leproma) invading almost the entire cornea. Marked vascularization. The process is asymptomatic and indolent. Many Hansen's bacilli are found in the corneal scraping.

6. Lepra maculo-anaesthetica. The process localizes in neuroglia of peripheral nerves, causing lepra claw of the hands. Ocular muscle paresis may occur.

PLATE XII   71

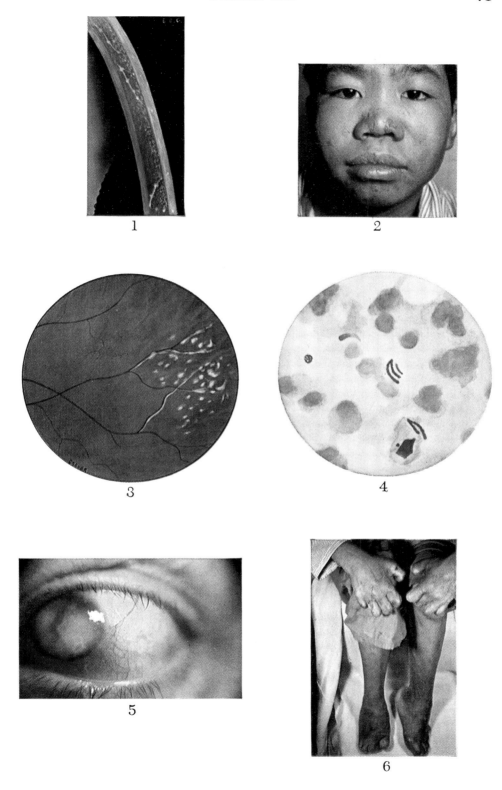

1

2

3

4

5

6

PLATE XIII

1. Infantile purulent conjunctivitis due to the gonococcus. *Neisseria gonorrhoeae* is the prime offender. Staphylococci, streptococci, or other bacteria may also be causative agents. The conjunctivitis occurs (usually in institutions) in girls aged 2 to 10 by contact with infected sources, human or environmental.

2A. Gonococcal ophthalmia neonatorum. General aspect. Note the abundant discharge and marked edema of lids. The examiner should protect his eyes (wearing glasses is best) from spurting pus when he opens the lids.

2B. Conjunctiva of same case. Infiltrated conjunctiva is rough and red, not as in staphylococcal or other infections (see page 16).

3. Morphologic characteristics of the gonococcus.

A. Original smear (gram stain). Smear morphology is more typical than in culture: gram-negative, kidney-shaped diplococci, usually seen within neutrophils. Cell response is mainly neutrophilic. Direct smear is needed, being sufficient for preliminary diagnosis.

B. Smear from young culture (gram stain). In older culture, gonococci autolyze and die rapidly, showing poorly stained, swollen, and irregular forms.

4. Gonococci in scraping (Giemsa stain). This shows turflike appearance within and at the edge of epithelial cells. May be found before the exudate smear is positive.

5. Fermentation reactions.

Glucose (dextrose): positive (yellow).

Maltose: negative (red).

6. Gonococci on chocolate agar. Colonies are round, mucoid, with irregular edges. (Growth more ready than on blood agar.)

PLATE XIII 73

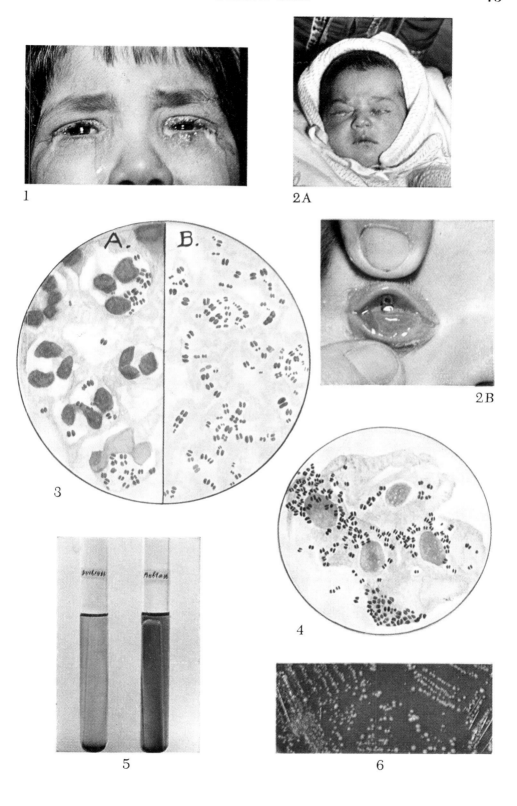

PLATE XIV

1. Keratitis (slit lamp view). Rare in meningococcal infections. A large area of the cornea is slightly and diffusely opaque, in which area are localized more extensive opacities. One deep vessel is demonstrated in the slit lamp beam.

2. Meningococci in original smear (gram stain). Kidney-shaped, intracellular, diplo-arranged meningococci, morphologically indistinguishable from gonococci.

3. Meningococci in smear from culture (gram stain). Meningococci autolyze and die, not as rapidly as gonococci. Note swollen, poorly stained forms.

4. Fermentation reactions.
   Maltose: positive (yellow).
   Glucose: positive (yellow).
   Sucrose: negative (red).

5. Oxidase test in culture on blood agar. Black spots show a positive oxidase reaction for all members of the *Neisseria* genus. By this test, neisseria can be identified in mixed culture.

PLATE XIV   75

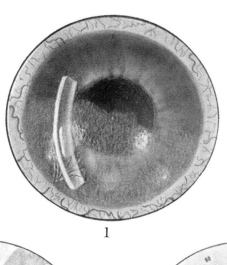

1

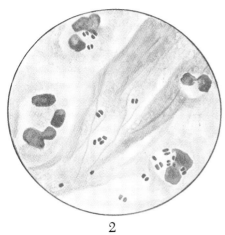

2

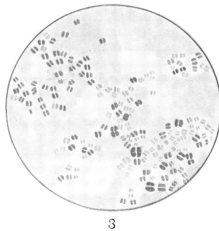

3

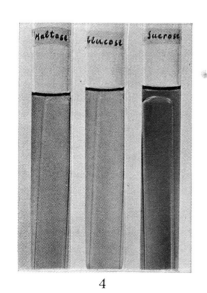

4

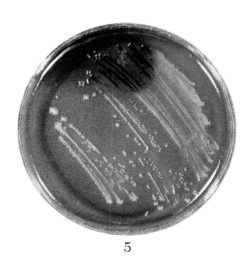

5

PLATE XV

1. *Neisseria catarrhalis* in original smear (methylene blue stain). Morphology is similar to that of the gonococcus and the meningococcus. Also can be found intracellularly.

2. *N. catarrhalis* in smear from culture (gram stain). Unlike *N. gonorrhoeae* and *N. meningitidis*, cocci are stable and regular in size and staining. No autolysis or degeneration is visible.

3. *N. catarrhalis* culture on blood agar.

    A. Original culture. Colonies are mucoid and semitransparent. Unlike *N. gonorrhoeae* and *N. meningitidis,* this organism is readily cultivated on ordinary media.

    B. Subculture.

4. Fermentation reactions.

    Glucose (dextrose): negative (red).

    Maltose: negative (red).

5. *N. catarrhalis* culture on plain agar shows abundant growth. This is the simplest way to distinguish *N. catarrhalis* from the gonococcus and the meningococcus, which do not grow on plain agar.

PLATE XV 77

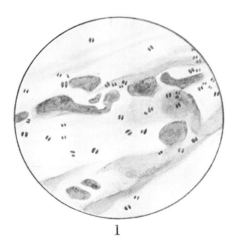

1

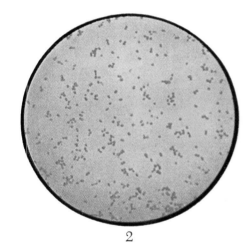

2

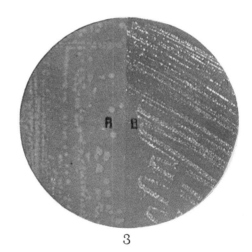

3

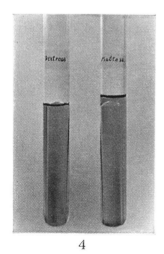

4

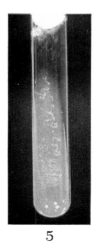

5

PLATE XVI

1. Angular blepharoconjunctivitis due to the Morax-Axenfeld diplobacillus *(Moraxella lacunata)*. A chronic process, it may last for years. Numerous diplobacilli are found, even in a mild, asymptomatic process. Without bacteriologic examination, the organism is easily overlooked (it may complicate intraocular surgery).

2. Central hypopyon keratitis due to the Morax-Axenfeld diplobacillus. Severe, purulent, destructive primary keratitis (without preceding angular blepharoconjunctivitis). This usually appears as a deep abscess and may have intact epithelium in the initial stage. Sterile hypopyon is present, indicating secondary iritis. When the abscess ulcerates, clean out the debris, then scrape the base for bacteriologic diagnosis.

3. Gram-negative diplobacilli in smears (gram stain).

   A. From culture on blood agar. Morphology of the Morax-Axenfeld diplobacillus usually changes rapidly. Note the pronounced polymorphism from long threads to coccobacilli. Some are club-shaped, resembling corynebacteria.

   B. Original smear from blepharoconjunctivitis exudate. Numerous gram-negative diplobacilli with square-shaped, plump, diplo or short chain appearance (thus distinguishable from other ophthalmic gram-negative bacilli). Also note exudate with many fibrin threads and only a few leukocytes. Direct smear is sufficient for diagnosis; several *C. xerosis* cells are present, illustrating symbiosis with the Morax-Axenfeld diplobacillus.

4. Morax-Axenfeld diplobacillus culture on Löffler's serum (grows rapidly). This medium is particularly needed to demonstrate liquefaction. Note the circumscribed pits (lacunae) typical for *Moraxella lacunata*. No actual colonies of *M. lacunata* are seen. Whitish colonies are *C. xerosis*.

5. Morax-Axenfeld diplobacillus original culture on blood agar (does not grow readily). Scanty, semitransparent, and slightly mucoid, resembling enteric groups. Important indications for differentiation are: moderate growth, without confluence or odor.

PLATE XVI 79

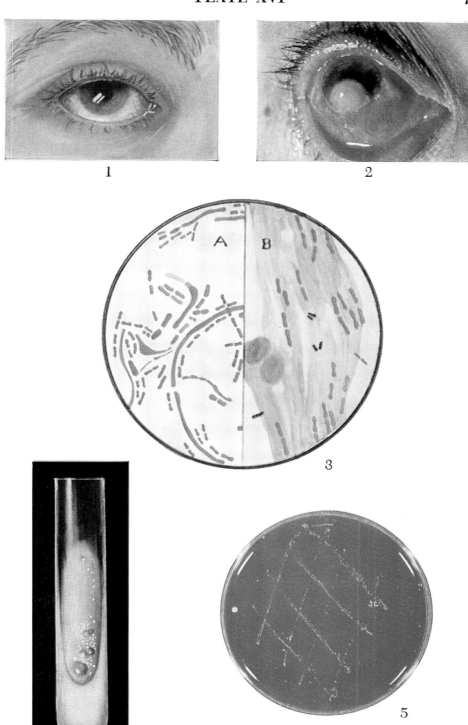

1

2

3

4

5

PLATE XVII

1. Corneal abscess (late stage) due to *Moraxella liquefaciens* (the Petit diplobacillus, probably a variant of *M. lacunata;* see page 90). This is a very destructive process, similar to that caused by *Moraxella lacunata* (see Plate XVI).

2. *M. liquefaciens* in smear and scraping (gram stain).

    A. From culture on blood agar. Gram-negative diplobacilli. No variation in morphology as in *M. lacunata.*

    B. Scraping from cornea (same case as 1, above). Diplobacilli similar to the Morax-Axenfeld diplobacillus. Note a few necrotic corneal epithelial cells.

3. *M. liquefaciens* culture on Löffler's serum. Liquefaction heavy and confluented. No definite pits (lacunae) as are characteristic for *M. lacunata.*

4. *M. liquefaciens* culture on blood agar. Diplobacilli grow readily. Colonies are semitransparent and slightly mucoid. No tendency to confluence, no odor.

PLATE XVII   81

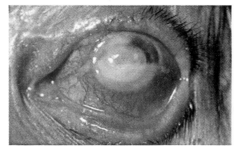

1

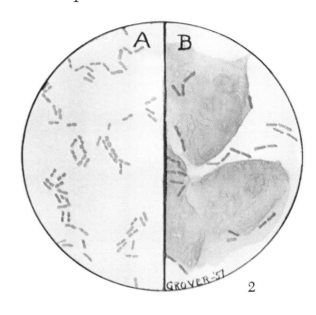

2

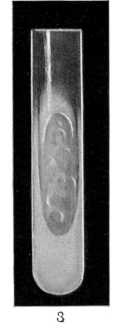

3

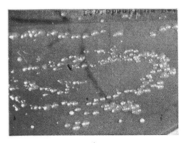

4

PLATE XVIII

1. Acute catarrhal conjunctivitis due to the Koch-Weeks bacillus *(Haemophilus aegyptius)*. Similar to pneumococcal conjunctivitis. Both have intensively hyperemic bulbar conjunctiva and a few petechiae. The discharge is mucopurulent and scanty, with excessive lacrimation. The cornea is rarely involved.

2. Picture demonstrates contagion of the Koch-Weeks bacillus. Family members developed similar acute conjunctivitis within two days.

3. Koch-Weeks bacillus in smears (gram stain).

A. From culture on blood agar. Gram-negative bacilli are minute, coccobacillary or slender. No characteristic arrangement. Often indistinguishable from the enteric group of bacilli. For diagnosis, cultural characteristics are needed.

B. Original smear of exudate. Slender gram-negative bacilli within leukocytes and between cells are shown. They are difficult to distinguish because of similar background color and minute size.

4. Koch-Weeks bacillus cultures on blood agar and on chocolate agar.

A. On blood agar. Colonies are tiny, translucent, with a dewdrop appearance. Satellite phenomenon: more luxuriant growth of bacilli around a single staphylococcal colony.

B. On chocolate agar, colonies are larger than on blood agar.

C. On blood agar.

5. Candle jar to grow culture in CO_2 atmosphere. The method is simple. Put plates at the bottom of the jar, light the candle, cover the jar. Incubate as usual.

6. Satellite phenomenon in original culture of blood agar. Zonular iridescent growth of Koch-Weeks bacilli around each of a few staphylococcal colonies.

PLATE XVIII   83

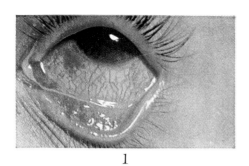

1

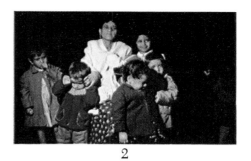

2

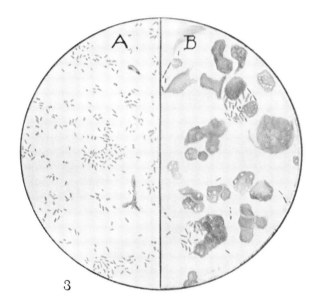

3

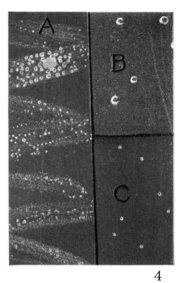

4

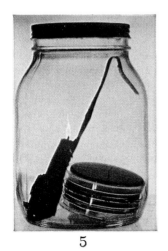

5

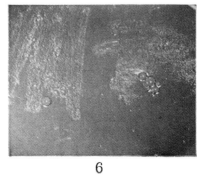

6

PLATE XIX

1. *Escherichia coli* and *Aerobacter aerogenes.* Smears from culture on blood agar.

    A. *E. coli.* Small, gram-negative bacilli. Pointed or rounded ends stain more intensively (polar stain). Morphologically indistinguishable from other enteric bacilli. Culture is important for diagnosis.

    B. *A. aerogenes.* May be distinguished from other enteric bacilli by its larger size and heavy capsule.

2. *E. coli* culture on MacConkey's agar. Colonies are uniformly red, large, and dull. This medium is better than blood agar for identification of *E. coli.*

3. Disk sensitivity test for *E. coli.* Single clear zone shows sensitivity of *E. coli* to Kantrex.

4. Blepharoconjunctivitis. Friedländer's bacillus *(Klebsiella pneumoniae)* found. Repeated isolation is important, as Friedländer's bacillus may be a contaminant.

5. *A. aerogenes* culture on blood agar. Colonies are easily recognized by their typical heavy, mucoid appearance. No hemolysis. (For details, see page 98.)

6. *E. coli* and *A. aerogenes* cultures on E.M.B. agar.

    E. coli: Has characteristic green metallic sheen (left half of plate).

    A. aerogenes: Colonies are dark red in center, colorless on periphery, larger and more mucoid than *E. coli* (right half of plate).

PLATE XIX

85

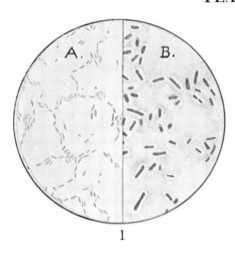

1

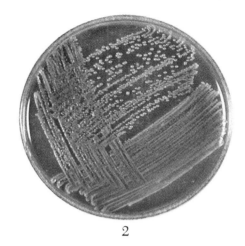

2

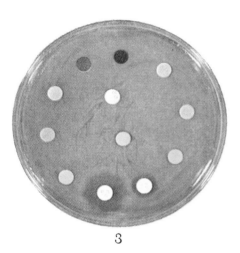

3

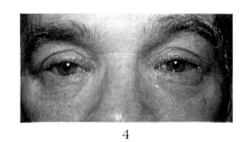

4

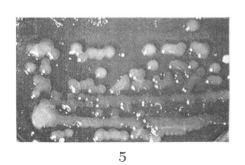

5

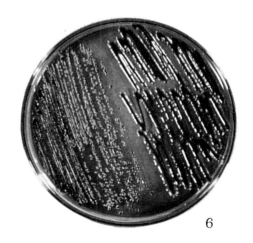

6

PLATE XX

1. Central hypopyon keratitis (caused by *Proteus vulgaris*). A destructive, abscesslike keratitis, usually associated with trauma. Repeated cultures are necessary, as *P. vulgaris* is often a contaminant.

2. *P. vulgaris* smear from blood agar culture. Small, gram-negative rods with pointed or rounded ends, showing polar stain. Indistinguishable from other gram-negative enteric bacilli.

3. *P. vulgaris* culture on blood agar. Note swarming growth over entire plate. The scratch crossing the circular waves was made to emphasize the diffuse, filmy growth. These waves indicate periodic growth. A putrid odor is detected at a distance.

4. Tests for differentiation of the enteric group.

Russell double sugar agar (left tube): indicates lactose-negative (butt is acid, slant is alkaline).

Simmon's citrate agar slant (middle tube): indicates citrate-negative.

SIM medium (right tube): indicates indol-positive and H_2S-positive (see page 97).

PLATE XX 87

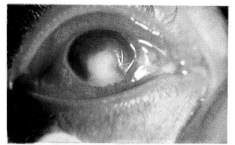

1

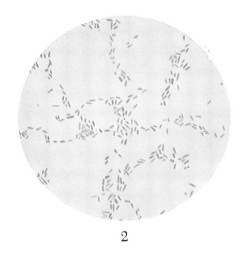

2

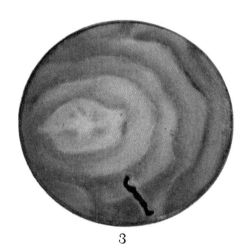

3

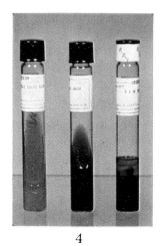

4

PLATE XXI

1. *Pseudomonas aeruginosa (Bacillus pyocyaneus)* smear from culture (gram stain). Small gram-negative rods (as are other enteric bacilli). Culture is necessary for diagnosis.

2. *Ps. aeruginosa* culture on blood agar. Colonies and surrounding medium are a dark greenish gray due to pigment production. The strong, sweet odor is an important diagnostic aid.

3. Central hypopyon keratitis due to *Ps. aeruginosa.* The process is characterized by severe and rapid necrosis, often resulting in perforation. Laboratory diagnosis followed by intensive therapy is urgent.

4. Bilateral lacrimal mucocele. This condition results from prolonged chronic dacryocystitis; an atonic sac with exudate is present. Mixed flora is usually found. This case was unusual, as a pure culture of *Ps. aeruginosa* was isolated.

5. Fluorescein solution. *Ps. aeruginosa* contaminates fluorescein solution readily, presenting a serious ophthalmologic problem.

6. Disk sensitivity test for *Ps. aeruginosa.* Sensitivity indicated by two zones of inhibition (the larger, polymyxin B; the narrower, streptomycin).

PLATE XXI

89

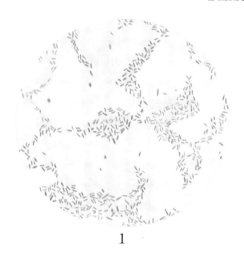

1

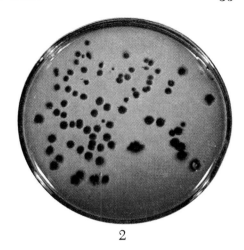

2

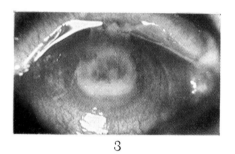

3

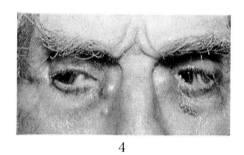

4

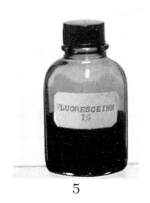

5

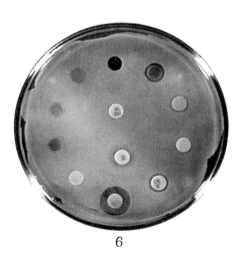

6

is necessary; a wooden toothpick will suffice. The applicator must be only dampened; any excess of the solution must be avoided. The cautery is applied only to the involved site, with care not to touch normal cornea. The cauterized tissue turns white, and this is an indication to stop the procedure immediately. A second treatment may be given in a day or two. Meanwhile, drops of 0.5 or 0.25 per cent zinc sulfate solution should be used three times a day. The physician should be aware that severe pain usually follows, in which case systemic pain medication is indicated. Sulfonamides, streptomycin, tetracyclines, or neomycin are used depending upon antibiotic sensitivity tests. Surgical procedures, including Saemisch's section, Sondermann's trephination, and delimiting keratotomy, have been used. These procedures may reduce the tension and bring additional antibodies from the secondary aqueous.

Recently, in our department, keratoplasty (lamellar or, in deep process, perforating) has been successful in saving the eye.

Enzymatic debridement with streptokinase, streptodornase, or, particularly, dornase can be effective.

Supportive measures, such as a good diet with vitamin B supplement, should be given, especially when the patient is alcoholic or otherwise debilitated.

Moraxella liquefaciens
(Diplobacillus of Petit)

In 1899, Petit isolated an organism from three cases of purulent keratitis. On the basis of clinical and laboratory evidence, he considered this to be a distinct entity, although it had some similarity to *M. lacunata*.

From a clinical point of view, he believed *M. lacunata* to be of low infectivity, able to cause only a mild process such as angular blepharoconjunctivitis. When the diplobacillus had sufficiently high virulence to cause a severe hypopyon keratitis, he called it the diplobacillus of Petit (now *Moraxella liquefaciens*).

While Petit found these two diplobacilli to be indistinguishable morphologically, he felt that their cultural characteristics were different. He declared that the Petit diplobacillus, unlike the Morax-Axenfeld diplobacillus, could grow on ordinary media and had the ability to liquefy Löffler's serum more effectively.

His views greatly affected our concept of diplobacillary keratitis. The name Petit was linked with virtually every case of diplobacillary keratitis. However, many cases of central hypopyon keratitis have been reported as being due to *M. lacunata*, and therefore much confusion has arisen. Later studies reveal that there is no serologic or cultural difference between the organisms isolated from both clinical entities. Various investigators have grown both organisms on ordinary media.

THE HAEMOPHILUS GENUS

The genus *Haemophilus* of the family *Brucellaceae* includes many members.

Haemophilus influenzae is the most important pathogen of this genus; it was described as the cause of influenza by Pfeiffer in 1893. Since that time many other members of the genus have been described, many of which are nonpathogenic. Among those pathogenic for man are *Haemophilus influenzae, Haemophilus ducreyi,* and *Haemophilus aegyptius* (the Koch-Weeks bacillus). *H. aegyptius,* strictly an ocular pathogen, is recognized by ophthalmologists as a species of the hemophilic group. Formerly, this organism was considered identical to *H. influenzae;* however, they are now regarded as two separate species.

Haemophilus aegyptius
(The Koch-Weeks Bacillus)

This bacillus was first described by Koch, when in 1884 he found it as a secondary invader in trachoma in Egypt. Independently, Weeks in 1886 described the same bacillus as the cause of epidemic acute conjunctivitis in New York. Since that time this type of conjunctivitis has been recognized along the coastlines of the United States and throughout Europe and Africa. It is very rare in Central America.

In Egypt, the Koch-Weeks bacillus is very common, hence the name *H. aegyptius.* It frequently causes an infection superimposed on trachoma; the entire process then resembles gonoblennorrhea.

Minton described epidemics of infective conjunctivitis in Iraq, Palestine, and Egypt. The epidemics usually occurred yearly (from May to August) among children. Ulceration of the cornea frequently complicated the conjunctivitis.

Morphology. Though typical in smear secretion, the organism is not easily found. The bacillus is minute, usually coccobacillary or slender gram-negative rod. The bacilli take a very pale stain from safranin (counter-stain by the gram method); carbolfuchsin gives a better result. There is no characteristic arrangement, and the organisms may appear singly, in pairs, short chains, or tangled masses. In smear secretion the bacilli are found free or intracellularly within the leukocytes and epithelial cells. Because of their small size they are adapted to an intracellular habitat. This can be better demonstrated in scrapings (Plate XVIII, 3B).

The morphology varies when the organism is cultured. The same strain can be so pleomorphic that it is difficult to recognize as the same organism. Wavy, curved, and very long filamentous forms develop in the culture (Plate XVIII, 3A). In young cultures on rich media, smooth (S) forms are encapsulated; the capsule is rarely found in an older culture.

A culture is necessary for diagnosis.

Culture.   Both *H. influenzae* and *H. aegyptius* require both the X and V factors. The V factor is found in vegetables. In animal tissue and yeast both factors are present. Both factors are also present in blood and are liberated from the blood cells by heating. Levinthal (brain-heart infusion agar with heated and filtered blood) and chocolate agar are ideal media. *Haemophilus* species also grow on the usual blood agar. An atmosphere of CO_2, as in a candle jar, favors growth (Plate XVIII, 5).

The colonies are tiny, glistening, translucent and pinpoint, with a dewdrop appearance (Plate XVIII, 4A). The pronounced sweet odor is of great diagnostic aid and leads one to search for the tiny colonies which might easily be overlooked.

The satellite phenomenon, seen in the presence of staphylococcic colonies, especially *S. aureus*, is another important characteristic. This phenomenon may also occur in the presence of other bacteria. A zone of iridescent growth of bacilli is seen around a staphylococcic colony. Here the bacillary colonies are larger than the others on the plate (Plate XVIII, 6). Sometimes the presence of a single staphylococcal colony may make diagnosis possible, since the bacilli may grow only around it, the plate being otherwise barren.

Antigenic Structure.   *H. aegyptius* and *H. influenzae* are closely related antigenically. The encapsulated forms of influenza bacilli have specific polysaccharide antigens, related to the capsule. Since these bacilli easily lose their capsule, their antigenic property is not stable. The majority of antigenic types are found among the virulent S strains. Six antigenic types are distinguished, a to f. Serologically and chemically the bacillary capsular polysaccharides resemble those of the pneumococci, and serologic cross reaction with pneumococcal antigens is common. The Quellung test for the antigenic typing of bacillus *H. influenzae* is identical with the pneumococcal test. Clinically there is similarity with acute Koch-Weeks conjunctivitis which is indistinguishable from pneumococcal conjunctivitis.

Pathogenesis.   Although *H. influenzae* has produced infection in laboratory animals, *H. aegyptius* is not usually pathogenic for them. These bacilli do not produce endotoxin, and their mode of disease production is unclear.

The encapsulated *H. influenzae* is virulent, producing in man a suppurative inflammation mainly in the respiratory tract. The organism is not now regarded as the cause of influenza, but rather as a secondary invader to primary infection caused by the influenza virus. Nevertheless, there is still controversy concerning its role in influenzal diseases.

Findings in the Eye.   The Koch-Weeks bacillus is the principal etiologic agent for acute mucopurulent conjunctivitis, which occurs mainly in the summer, predominantly in southern climates.[33] The exudate is mucoid in nature and not usually abundant. There is a great deal of associated lacrimation. The conjunctivitis becomes purulent if there is poor hygiene or low resistance. Clinically it is similar to pneumococcal conjunctivitis and is characterized by involvement of the bulbar conjunctiva, which exhibits a typical cyanotic redness. Small hemorrhages may occur, mainly in the upper bulbar conjunctiva (Plate XVIII, 1), but these are not as prominent as they seem in pneumococcal conjunctivitis. Enlargement and tenderness of the preauricular glands occur. The bacilli are not easy to find in the secretion because of their small size and red color, which is hard to distinguish from the red background. A scraping from the bulbar conjunctiva may reveal the organism even prior to its appearance in the secretion. This infection is contagious and is usually epidemic, particularly in families, schools, or other institutions (Plate XVIII, 2).

Secondary corneal involvement is unusual in our experience. These bacilli have no affinity for corneal avascular tissue. However, in the tropics, corneal complications are not uncommon and may occur elsewhere. The author has described four cases of severe keratitis complicating acute conjunctivitis due to Koch-Weeks bacilli. This was observed in the 1927 epidemic of conjunctivitis at Dniepropetrovsk in the Ukraine. The cases of keratitis were perhaps due to the greater virulence of the bacteria seen in this particular epidemic or to lowered resistance of these patients. Primary central corneal keratitis without preceding conjunctivitis is unknown.

Severe pseudomembranous conjunctivitis sometimes occurs in newborn children.

Cases of endophthalmitis caused by this bacillus have been occasionally recorded.

Koch-Weeks bacilli are not infrequently found in the pus from an infected lacrimal sac or in the secretion of the meibomian glands.

Treatment. The bacilli are susceptible to streptomycin, the tetracyclines, and sulfonamides. Topical treatment suffices for the treatment of the conjunctivitis.

Haemophilus ducreyi

This small gram-negative bacillus was described by Ducrey in 1889 as the cause of soft chancre (chancroid). The bacillus has many morphologic and biologic characteristics in common with H. influenzae. It has similar growth requirements, except that it needs only one of the growth factors, X, in the blood medium. Bacteriologic isolation of the bacillus from clinical material is very difficult, as it is usually associated with numerous other pyogenic bacteria.

For diagnosis of chancroid the skin test with killed culture of H. ducreyi bacilli is used. Ocular infections due to Ducrey's bacillus are extremely rare.

SMALL GRAM-NEGATIVE BACILLI

These are the smallest of all bacilli, having an imperfect inner structure. Hence most of them are adapted to an intracellular habitat.

Laboratory identification of *Brucella* and *Pasteurella* is difficult. Strictly aseptic precautions are required because of high infectivity. Diagnosis is usually established by trained workers in specially equipped laboratories.

Bacilli of this group are rarely found in the eye. They are usually studied in detail by general bacteriologists. A few principal characteristics will be discussed briefly.

Brucella Genus

Members of this genus are classified according to their hosts, goats, cattle, and swine: *Br. melitensis, Br. abortus,* and *Br. suis.* The identification is not distinct; they are sometimes considered variants of the same strain. All three, particularly *Br. melitensis,* may cause brucellosis in man. *Br. melitensis* was isolated from cases among military personnel on Malta, hence the popular name Malta fever. Milk and urine are the main sources of infection.

Man is highly susceptible to brucella, but the infection is frequently subclinical. The only positive diagnosis is the isolation of the organism from the blood or urine. Other tests such as the skin test and the agglutination tests may be used as aids in the diagnosis but never in themselves assure the diagnosis. Clinical manifestations are divided into three groups: acute, subacute, and chronic. The latter may last from 1 to 20 years.

Laboratory Studies. Brucella bacilli are found in direct secretion, are typically gram-negative, and found within reticuloendothelial cells. Being tiny, the bacilli may be confused with intracellular granules.

Diagnosis is more successful with cultivation. The brucella bacilli grow on many media; *Br. abortus* requires CO_2 tension; Brewer's medium can be satisfactorily used. Identification of the species requires numerous additional factors.

Diagnosis is often made by ascertaining the agglutination titer of the patient's serum. Because the test is often positive in a healthy person, diagnosis of brucellosis should not be made unless the titer is at least 1:500. Usually titers of 1:60 and up indicate infection.

The patient's blood, or material from the lesions, or both, are used for laboratory investigation.

Findings in the Eye. Brucellosis of the eye is secondary to systemic brucellosis, and primary invasion is almost unknown.

Involvements of the eye vary geographically.[12] They are rare, although in some countries they may be more frequent. When the eye is involved, the inner eye is predominantly affected, particularly the uvea. The process is usually the granulomatous type and may involve the entire uvea. In iritis, nodules occur at the pupillary border.

Nummular keratitis associated with brucellosis has been reported by Woods. He also produced this keratitis experimentally by inoculation with brucella, and has suggested the term "brucella nummular keratitis,"

In Mexico, where brucellosis is widespread, the optic nerve is most frequently affected. Therefore, any patient with pathology of the optic nerve is routinely investigated for brucella.

Other ocular complications of systemic brucellosis are: dacryocystitis and panophthalmitis, the latter appearing similar to that caused by the tubercle bacillus.

Treatment. Chlortetracycline, chloramphenicol, and oxytetracycline give a striking result in treatment of brucellosis. Adding sulfadiazine and streptomycin may be helpful. Fever therapy is highly recommended. Vaccine therapy has been tried.

Pasteurella Genus

The identification of this broad group is indistinct. These bacilli are associated with various animal hosts. The species most frequently affecting man are: *Past. pestis, Past. pseudotuberculosis,* and *Past. tularensis. Past. multocida,* isolated from deer, is also pathogenic for man.

Past. pestis is a primary cause of disease in rats and various wild rodents. When transmitted to man it produces plague, which without therapy is invariably fatal. Sometimes the organisms are so highly virulent that a single bacillus can be lethal.

The bacilli are short, ovoid, plump, gram-negative rods. Many media are used to grow them, but blood agar plates are suitable for primary isolation.

Ocular diseases due to *Past. pestis* are almost unknown.

Past. pseudotuberculosis produces disease in birds and various kinds of animals. Extremely rarely it may be transmitted to man.

Past. tularensis is of interest in ophthalmology as a cause of Parinaud's oculoglandular syndrome. These bacilli are parasites of hares and wild rodents. The name tularemia is from Tulare, a county in California where the disease was first identified. It can be transmitted to man by skinning or eating animals infected with *Past. tularensis.* Usually generalized, characterized by fever and adenopathy, the infection spreads via the blood to parenchymatous organs, as does the process due to brucellae and other pasteurellae. The disease may be fatal. Sometimes it is localized at the portal of entry, and it is usually associated with regional adenopathy.

Laboratory Studies. Morphologically the bacilli are pleomorphic, tiny, usually coccobacillary, sometimes encapsulated, gram-negative.

Past. tularensis does not grow on ordinary culture media. However, egg yolk medium or blood glucose cystine agar is generally used for cultivation; minute grayish white colonies develop. Brewer's medium, especially with fresh blood added, can also be satisfactorily employed.

Agglutination is a valuable diagnostic test for tularemia. The test is considered positive when agglutination occurs in serum diluted 1:80 or higher.

Findings in the Eye. The eye may be primarily affected through the conjunctiva, which is more vulnerable than the skin. The incubation period is about three days, and onset is sudden. The process is prolonged—about four weeks—is mainly unilateral, and is characterized by scattered, small, yellow, necrotic ulcers or nodules. The tarsal conjunctiva of the lower lid is primarily affected; however, the upper can be involved (but not the bulbar). The infection is accompanied by fever and enlargement of the preauricular and submaxillary glands (oculoglandular Parinaud's syndrome). Suppuration of the glands, requiring an operation, is a frequent sequela. Nodular lesions resembling phlyctenules may occur rarely on the bulbar conjunctiva. This is characteristically painful. Although ocular tularemia is rare, it is more frequent in France;[7,43] 112 cases were reported there in 1949-1950. These were predominantly the granulomatous type, followed by ulceration. Systemic symptoms were usually absent, but Parinaud's syndrome was constantly present.

Treatment. There is no specific treatment. The most effective is streptomycin. However, broad-spectrum antibiotics in the early stages may be effective. A hot compress gives comfort.

ENTERIC BACTERIA

This encompasses a wide group of gram-negative bacilli, saprophytic and pathogenic, found in the intestinal canal. The pathogens are shigellae or salmonellae; although bacilli of the coliform group are a part of its normal flora they may become pathogenic. The *Pseudomonas* and *Proteus* genera, related to the coliform group, are also discussed.

The pathogens characteristically fail to ferment lactose. Hence, the lactose fermentation test is generally used as a preliminary one for differentiation of these enteric pathogens from nonpathogens.

The nonpathogenic enteric bacilli are not uncommon etiologic agents for infections of the genitourinary or respiratory tracts, and of the eye or other parts of the body. Injured tissue is more easily invaded. These bacilli have a number of common characteristics, a brief description of which may simplify diagnosis. They are morphologically indistinguishable, and their identification in smear is impossible. A culture is necessary. All are gram-negative bacilli, varying in size from short, coccobacillary forms to long filamentous ones, with rounded or pointed ends. Capsules are not constantly present except in the genus *Klebsiella*. There is nothing characteristic in their arrangement; they may be present singly, in pairs, short chains, or in groups.

All members of these groups grow readily on simple, ordinary media, even at room temperature. Colonies are semitranslucent and mucoid on solid media, with a tendency to become confluent. Many members are actively motile, and they all produce a strong odor.

They ferment a wide range of carbohydrates. The positive lactose fermentation differentiates most of these bacilli from the pathogens (*Shigella* and *Salmonella* genera) which show negative lactose fermentation tests. Their complex antigenic structures result in serologic interrelationships between different groups and species.

Outside the intestinal canal these bacilli may produce a purulent type of inflammation; endotoxin is probably an important factor. The enteric bacilli are found often in normal flora of various mucosa or as secondary invaders because the excessive use of antibiotics causes imbalanced flora. Their etiologic role can be determined only by repeated cultivation.

Coliform Bacteria or Colon-Aerogenes Group
(Genera *Escherichia, Aerobacter,* and *Klebsiella*)

Escherichia and *Aerobacter* (*aerogenes* and *cloacae*) are closely related, hence their distinction is not easy; however, it is particularly necessary for purposes of sanitation control. Finding *E. coli* in milk or water proves fecal contamination, but the presence of *Aerobacter* usually does not so indicate. Hence, many detailed differential tests have been devised to distinguish the organisms.

The organisms exhibit some morphologic and cultural differences, such as: the capsule is more prominent and colonies are more mucoid in *Aerobacter aerogenes* than in *E. coli* (Plate XIX, 1), but these are not constant and are not very significant. Biochemical characteristics are more important for differentiation. *E. coli* produces indole, the methyl red test is positive, the Voges-Proskauer test is negative, and there is no utilization of citrate. On the contrary, *Aerobacter* does not produce indole, the methyl red test is negative, and the Voges-Proskauer and citrate tests are positive. These differences may be demonstrated in the following media:

E.M.B. (*Eosin Methylene Blue*) *Agar.* *E. coli* colonies are small and dry, with a characteristic green metallic sheen. *Aerobacter* colonies are large, mucoid, and dark red in the center though colorless on the periphery (Plate XIX, 6).

MacConkey's Medium. *E. coli* colonies are usually large, dry and bright pink. *Aerobacter* colonies are moist and mucoid, and the center is usually red, with the periphery colorless.

Simmons' Citrate Agar. *E. coli* does not utilize citrate and there is no color change in the medium. *Aerobacter* utilizes citrate and changes the medium from green to blue.

SIM Medium. *E. coli* is indole-positive; *Aerobacter* is indole-negative.

E. coli and *Aerobacter* show similarity in their pathogenicity and in their resistance to antibiotics. Hence in ophthalmology, distinct differentiation, which is rather complex, has more theoretical than practical interest.

Antigenic Structure. This is complex and varied. *E. coli* has numerous flagellar, capsular, and somatic antigens. Two types of antigens are best known: O, a somatic antigen of the bacterial body, and H, a flagellar antigen. A capsular antigen, K, has recently been recognized. Most strains of *E. coli* are motile.

Pathogenicity and Pathology. Pathogenicity of *E. coli* is due to endotoxins and to the flagellar and capsular antigens. *E. coli* and less frequently, *Aerobacter*, may cause infections of the eye, gallbladder, the urinary or respiratory tracts, or others. The usual type of inflammation is purulent, with grayish green exudate. Any one of these infections can result in toxemia. Septicemia rarely develops in the newborn.

Findings in the Eye. *E. coli* seldom causes ocular infections.[6, 10] It more often occurs as a secondary invader, and only repeated positive cultures can prove its causative role. It may be found in a small percentage of normal conjunctivas, especially in persons with intestinal ailments or following prolonged use of antibiotics.

In the conjunctiva, the bacillus has been described rarely as a cause of purulent ophthalmia in newborn infants. It may also cause pseudomembranous conjunctivitis in adult persons. Hypopyon keratitis due to *E. coli* is uncommon; lack of affinity for corneal tissue is suggested (Vaughan). This severe hypopyon keratitis in the form of a deep abscess has been personally observed at Bellevue Hospital. It is usually associated with corneal damage in debilitated patients.

The organism has also rarely caused panophthalmitis, cellulitis of the orbit, and dacryocystitis.

Treatment. The susceptibility of *E. coli* to antibiotics varies greatly, and sensitivity tests must be performed. The organisms may resist all antibiotics. Neomycin and polymyxin usually give a better effect than the other antibiotics. Wide-spectrum antibiotic treatment is more effective in severe cases such as hypopyon keratitis. In our laboratory, sensitivity of *E. coli* to Kantrex has been demonstrated (Plate XIX, 3). The pupil should be kept dilated in keratitis. If conjunctivitis alone is present, local treatment suffices.

Klebsiella Genus

This is a genus of coliform bacteria which, though closely related to *E. coli,* shows a more marked capsule and heavy mucoid growths. The organisms present ill-defined bacteriology and are classified mainly on the basis of the clinical picture. The varying nomenclature applied to klebsiella in association with certain diseases is a source of confusion.

The bacillus found in patients with pneumonia is usually called *Klebsiella pneumoniae* (Friedländer's bacillus). In urologic practice it is designated as *Aerobacter.* Hence, this group is sometimes called *Klebsiella-Aerobacter.* The name *Klebsiella* is constantly applied to the clinical entities ozena and rhinoscleroma (*K. ozaenae* and *K. rhinoscleromatis*). The etiologic role of these bacilli is questioned, although they are found in the above diseases.

Morphology. Morphologically the organisms are distinguished from the other enteric bacilli by their heavy capsules, fat appearance, shortness (Plate XIX, 1B), and the fact that they can occur as coccobacilli. The bacilli are a very faint pink with gram stain, although from an old culture the stain may not take at all. The bacilli are arranged singly, in short chains, or as diplobacilli.

Culture. Klebsiella grow easily on simple media, as do all other enteric bacilli. They have a variety of cultural characteristics in association with the source of the culture. Nevertheless, the heavy mucoid appearance and a tendency to confluence is a common and distinguishing characteristic of all klebsiella and aerobacter (Plate XIX, 5). The mucoid consistency may be demonstrated by touching the colony with a loop; strings of material hang on the loop as it is removed. These organisms do not develop a characteristic odor and show no hemolysis. The culture is recognized usually without difficulty.

Findings in the Eye. *K. pneumoniae* may occur in the normal conjunctiva, but it is rarely the etiologic agent for a pathologic condition; however, a few ocular infections have been reported. These are keratitis in the form of a ring abscess, metastatic orbital abscess, dacryocystitis, pseudomembranous conjunctivitis of the newborn, even keratomalacia in infants. A pure culture of *K. pneumoniae* was isolated in our laboratory in a case of acute blepharoconjunctivitis (Plate XIX, 4).

The contact transference of the bacilli to the conjunctiva may occur sporadically in ozena. They may play a role in ocular infection, particularly of injured tissue. Their etiologic role can be decided only if the bacilli are plentiful in the conjunctival secretions, as they are usually secondary invaders.

Treatment. The klebsiella bacilli are sensitive to most antibiotics except penicillin; the sensitivity test helps determine the choice. Since resistant strains appear rapidly, an antibiotic is best introduced together with sulfonamide, or two types of antibiotic should be used simultaneously.

Pseudomonas Genus

This is a broad group of bacilli distributed widely in soil and water.

Pseudomonas aeruginosa (*Bacillus pyocyaneus*) is a pathogen for man, and while saprophytic in the intestinal canal, it may become virulent outside.

In normal intestinal flora, *Ps. aeruginosa* multiplies rapidly if the coliform bacilli are suppressed, especially after prolonged treatment with antibiotics.

Morphologically *Ps. aeruginosa* is indistinguishable from the other gram-negative enteric bacilli, and diagnosis in smear secretion is impossible (Plate XXI, 1).

Culture. The culture, besides its general characteristics, has a few distinguishing features. It produces two types of pigment: pyocyanin and fluorescein. Both pigments develop best at room temperature during daylight and in a fluid medium; in the latter, the pigment may best be demonstrated after shaking the tube to increase oxidation.

The colonies on blood agar are dark greenish gray, and because of pigment production the surrounding medium becomes bluish green (Plate XXI, 2). Aged colonies have a gummy consistency, and vigorous scraping may be necessary to obtain a suitable specimen.

A strong, sweet, haylike odor is produced by *Ps. aeruginosa.*

On the basis of the cultural characteristics *Ps. aeruginosa* can usually be recognized without further identification.

It has recently been shown that *Ps. aeruginosa* may be highly bactericidal for other bacteria. This is possibly due to the lytic action of the pyocyanease or of the pigment.

Pathology. *Ps. aeruginosa* was first isolated by Gessard in 1882 from "blue pus." The organism, outside the intestinal canal, is a common finding in the purulent inflammation of wounds and in the urinary tract. It is also found in infants' summer diarrhea and in inflammation of the middle and external ears. In the eye, *Ps. aeruginosa* causes the most destructive hypopyon keratitis. A septicemia complicated by endocarditis may occur. The bacilli cause patchy necrosis and ulceration on the skin. Nevertheless, in many of these conditions they may be only secondary invaders. *Ps. aeruginosa* has been isolated from the pharynx in cases of agranulocytic angina; however, the etiologic agent of the neutropenia is uncertain. The organisms' pathogenicity may be proved in all these infections by inoculation of a culture into a rabbit cornea; if the organisms are virulent, an abscess develops.

Ps. aeruginosa is much more virulent in the tropics and produces a systemic disease resembling typhoid fever.

Burns and Rhodes reported pseudomonas infection as a cause of death in four premature infants.

Findings in the Eye. Ocular disease due to *Ps. aeruginosa,* while uncommon, may be of great severity.[28, 44]

A primary conjunctivitis seldom occurs. A membranous type of conjunctivitis, usually secondary to keratitis, is reported.[30] In our case of bilateral lacrimal mucocele, a pure culture of *Ps. aeruginosa* was isolated (Plate XXI, 4).

Hypopyon keratitis sometimes occurs; this may be abscesslike (Plate XXI, 3) or in the form of a ring abscess or serpiginous ulcer.[49] The process is characterized by a rapid course and necrosis, which may result in perforation within 24 hours. The only possibility of saving the eye is prompt recognition and early treatment. Signs and symptoms aiding early diagnosis are:

1. There is nearly always a history of corneal injury, most often by a foreign body.

2. In approximately 9 out of 10 cases there is a history of recent ocular therapy or examination in which fluorescein was used.

3. The chief ocular and early symptom is pain, occurring one to three days following the corneal insult. At the time, there are usually signs of corneal opacity and infiltration; ulceration soon follows.

4. Epidemiology. The vast majority of cases appear in minor, sporadic epidemics which can usually be traced to a single source of contamination.

Summary. To establish an early diagnosis, pyocyaneous keratitis must be suspected in all cases that exhibit the following triad—1, foreign body; 2, local therapy; and 3, ocular pain—one to three days after a corneal insult.

The eye infections ranged from conjunctivitis through corneal abscess to endophthalmitis, orbital cellulitis, and septicemia. Fisher and Allen showed in experiments that *Ps. aeruginosa* elaborates an enzyme, called protease, which has a proteolytic activity against collagen of the cornea. Therefore, the corneal process is rapid and necrotic. However, in all severe infections the host resistance is most important.

In ophthalmology, the ease and frequency with which fluorescein solution may be contaminated with *Ps. aeruginosa* presents a serious problem. The search for rapidly acting preservatives is essential. The obvious answer to the problem is the use of fluorescein strips. However, if the solution must be used, every precaution should be taken to ensure its sterility.

Treatment. Unfortunately, most antimicrobial agents have proved ineffective.[35] However, the infection responds best to polymyxin B (Plate XXI, 6) and E, especially if administered early. An excellent result following prolonged therapy with subconjunctival polymyxin B in a dosage of 10 to 40 mg every two or three days has been reported. Coly-mycin, a new drug, is said to be the best therapeutic agent thus far for pseudomonas. Clinical observation is in process. In severe infection, shotgun therapy with antibiotics is advisable, with instillation of atropine to prevent iritis.

Prophylaxis. It is important to find and eliminate the source of contamination. All patients who have been exposed to the contaminant should receive local polymyxin therapy within three days.

Proteus Genus

The organisms of the *Proteus* genus have been known since the earliest days of bacteriology. Proteus bacilli, widely distributed in nature, exist as saprophytes in putrefying animal and vegetable matter. The bacilli rapidly decompose proteins and carbohydrates.

Proteus vulgaris, Proteus morganii, and *Proteus rettgeri* are of medical interest. *P. vulgaris* and *P. morganii* are usually saprophytic inhabitants of the intestinal canal. However, *P. morganii* has sometimes been a cause of summer diarrhea of children. Both may cause infection outside the canal.

Morphologically the organisms (Plate XX, 2) are indistinguishable from the other gram-negative bacilli (see page 96).

Culture. Cultural characteristics of proteus organisms are most significant for diagnosis. The ability to swarm on a solid medium, because of their active motility, is their most distinguishing feature. A uniform layer of spreading growth develops over the whole surface; the thin film is hard to see and may be overlooked. Scratching with a loop helps reveal the diffuse, filmy growth. The swarming growth often shows rippling waves moving either in one direction or in concentric rings, indicating periodic extensions of the growth (Plate XX, 3). Proteus bacilli produce a very strong odor of decay, easily detected at a distance. The bacilli may be recognized by these typical cultural characteristics. However, in atypical cases, several special tests are needed (Plate XX, 4). The positive urease test is most important.

Proteus bacilli frequently occur in mixed culture, swarming over the entire plate. They may mask the growth of organisms responsible for the infection. Therefore, narcotics such as chloral hydrate or morphine are used to inhibit spread of the proteus.

Antigenic Structure. There are two main antigens, H (flagellar) produced by motile proteus, and O (somatic) by nonmotile proteus. Certain strains of proteus called X have been isolated from the urine of patients with typhus fever, and the serum of the patient after four days agglutinated strains designated X19 and X2. Since the antigens are located in the bodies of nonmotile bacilli, they have been named OX19 and OX2. Agglutination of these strains by sera of patients with rickettsial infections is known as the Weil-Felix reaction. A positive Weil-Felix action has also been reported in trachoma.

Pathology. Proteus bacilli are usually found as secondary invaders in wounds. Nevertheless they are responsible for several suppurative processes in man, such as urinary infection and cystitis. Numerous proteus bacilli have been encountered in infantile diarrhea.

Findings in the Eye. Proteus, in the eye, is mainly a secondary contaminant. Since proteus bacilli may be contaminants of the culture medium, it is absolutely necessary to repeat the culture several times. Only then can the etiologic role of proteus be established.

Disease of the eye due to *P. vulgaris* is rare. However, recent reports indicate that it has a higher pathogenicity for the eye than has been suggested.[11] Proteus has been isolated from cases of severe keratitis similar to those caused by *Ps. aeruginosa*. A similar case from Bellevue Hospital is shown in Plate XX, 1. The process is usually rapid and destructive and can result in perforation of the cornea. This keratitis most commonly occurs in older persons, after injury. Endophthalmitis caused by proteus and panophthalmitis in premature infants have also been reported.

Proteus bacilli are sometimes found in conjunctivitis, dacryocystitis, and in some postoperative infections.

Treatment.   The same problem is present as with other gram-negative bacilli. *P. vulgaris* is not responsive to most antibiotics. In severe infections, shotgun therapy is recommended. Neomycin is the most active antibiotic. Streptomycin, Chloromycetin, and Neosporin have been successfully used.

REFERENCES

1. Ainslie, D.   Treatment of corneal infection with *Ps. pyocyanea* by subconjunctival injection of polymyxin E, Brit. J. Ophth., 37:336, 1953.
2. Allen, J. H., and Erdman, G. L.   Meningococcic keratoconjunctivitis, Am. J. Ophth., 29:721, 1946.
3. Armstrong, S. H., Jr., and Irons, E. N.   Physiological considerations of ACTH and cortisone therapy with reference to ophthalmology, Arch. Ophth., 45:251, 1951.
4. Axenfeld, T.   Über die chronische Diplobacillenconjunctivitis, Zentralbl. Bakt., 21:1, 1897.
5. Baraff, A. A. A.   Gonorrheal ophthalmia neonatorum, Illinois M. J., 87:249, 1945.
6. Berens, C., and Nilson, E. L.   Ocular conditions associated with coliform bacteria, Arch. Ophth., 26:816, 1941.
7. Brini, A., and Muller, J.   Oculo-glandular tularemia and the conjunctivitis of Parinaud (abstract), Am. J. Ophth., 35:159, 1952.
8. Burns, R. P., and Rhodes, D. M.   Pseudomonas eye infection as a cause of death in premature infants, Arch. Ophth., 65:517, 1961.
9. Cassady, J. V.   Pseudomonas corneal ulceration, Am. J. Ophth., 48:741, 1959.
10. Clark, G., and Locatcher-Khorazo, D.   Corneal ulcer produced by *Aerobacter aerogenes*, Arch. Ophth., 45:165, 1951.
11. Crabb, A. M., Fielding, I. L., and Ormsby, H. L.   *Bacillus proteus* endophthalmitis, Am. J. Ophth., 43:86, 1957.
12. Cremona, A. C.   Ocular manifestations of human brucellosis (abstract), Am. J. Ophth., 37:320, 1954.
13. de Roetth, A., Jr.   Annual reviews: Ophthalmic pharmacology and toxicology (prophylaxis of ophthalmia neonatorum), Arch. Ophth., 62:324, 1959.
14. Duke-Elder, W. S.   A text-book of Ophthalmology, St. Louis, C. V. Mosby Co., 1946, vol. 2.
15. Elliot, A. J., Chamberlain, W. P., Jr., and Givner, I.   Diplobacillus of Petit in corneal ulceration, Arch. Ophth., 25:280, 1941.
16. Fedukowicz, H., and Horwich, H.   The gram-negative diplobacillus in hypopyon keratitis, Arch. Ophth., 49:202, 1953.
17. ——— Wise, G. N., and Zaret, M. M.   Toxic conjunctivitis due to antibiotics, Am. J. Ophth., 40:849, 1955.
18. Fisher, E., Jr., and Allen, J. H.   Mechanism of corneal destruction by pseudomonas proteases, Am. J. Ophth., 46(Part 2):249, 1958.
19. Fox, J. E., and Lowbury, E. J. L.   Immunity to *Pseudomonas pyocyanea* in man, J. Path. & Bact., 65:519, 1953.
20. Givner, I.   *Neisseria catarrhalis* endophthalmitis, Am. J. Ophth., 32:699, 1949.
21. Horwich, H., and Fedukowicz, H.   Variation in Morax-Axenfeld diplobacillus, Arch. Ophth., 54:580, 1955.
22. Kahaner, J. R., and Lanou, W. W.   Exogenous meningococcic conjunctivitis, New York J. Med., 45:1687, 1945.
23. Kaivonen, M.   Comparative tests on the bactericidal effect of certain antiseptics and antibiotics, Acta ophth., 36:546, 1958.
24. Koch, R.   II. Bericht über die thätigkeit der deutschen Cholerakommission in Aegypten und Ostindien, Wien. med. Wchnschr., 33:1548, 1883.
25. Koenig, M. G., and Kaye, D.   Enterococcal endocarditis, Surv. Ophth., 6:248, 1961.

26. Lewis, P. M.   Ocular complications of meningococcic meningitis, Am. J. Ophth., 23:617, 1940.

27. ———   Penicillin in gonococcic conjunctivitis: its use in 30 cases compared with the sulfonamides in 173 cases, Am. J. Ophth., 29:694, 1946.

28. MacDonald, M.   *Ps. pyocyaneus* eye infection, Brit. J. Ophth., 37:370, 1953.

29. Mangiaracine, A. B., and Pollen, A.   Meningococcic conjunctivitis, Arch. Ophth., 31:284, 1944.

30. McCulloch, J. C.   Origin and pathogenicity of *Pseudomonas pyocyanea* in conjunctival sac, Arch. Ophth., 29:924, 1943.

31. McMeel, J. W., Wood, R. M., and Senterfit, L. B.   Effect of polymyxin B sulfate on pseudomonas corneal ulcers, Arch. Ophth., 66:646, 1961.

32. Meleney, F. L., and Prout, G. R., Jr.   Some laboratory and clinical observations on Coly-mycin (Colistin) with particular reference to pseudomonas infection, Surv. Ophth., 6:433, 1961.

33. Minton, J.   Eye diseases in the East, Brit. J. Ophth., 29:19, 1945.

34. Mitsui, Y., Hinokuma, S., and Tananka, C.   Etiology of angular conjunctivitis, Am. J. Ophth., 34:1579, 1951.

35. Moorman, L. T., and Harbert, F.   Treatment of Pseudomonas corneal ulcers, Arch. Ophth., 53:345, 1955.

36. Norn, M. S.   A quantitative method for studying the cytology of the conjunctiva, Acta ophth., 36:502, 1958.

37. Odegaard, K.   Conjunctivitis purulenta with keratitis caused by *Neisseria intracellularis*, Acta ophth., 21:295, 1944.

38. Oeding, P.   Diplobacillus liquefaciens of Petit isolated from a patient with ulcus serpens corneae, Acta ophth., 24:159, 1946.

39. Paraipan, C.   Pneumococcic corneal ulcer healed in 24 hours with penicillin, Am. J. Ophth., 30:475, 1947.

40. Rapis, G. B.   Phenomenon of chromatic "fatigue" in patients with brucellosis, Vestnik oftal., 73:31, 1960.

41. Reid, R. D., and Bronstein, L. H.   Meningococcic conjunctivitis, J.A.M.A., 124:703, 1944

42. Rodger, F. C.   Eye diseases in African children, Brit. J. Ophth., 42:336, 1958.

43. Rosenthal, J. N.   Oculoglandular tularemia (abstract), Am. J. Ophth., 34:163, 1951.

44. Spencer, W. H.   *Pseudomonas aeruginosa* infections of the eye, California Med., 79:438, 1953.

45. Suie, T., Blatt, M. M., Havener, W. H., Sroufe, S. A., and Balstad, P.   Bacterial corneal ulcers, Am. J. Ophth., 48:775, 1959.

46. Theodore, F. H., and Kost, P. F.   Meningococcic conjunctivitis, Arch. Ophth., 31:245, 1944.

47. ———   The classification and treatment of allergies of the conjunctiva, Am. J. Ophth., 36:1689, 1953.

48. Vaughan, D. G., Jr.   Corneal ulcers, Surv. Ophth., 3:203, 1958.

49. Williams, R. K., Hench, M. E., and Guerry, DuP., III.   Pyocyaneus ulcer, Am. J. Ophth., 37:538, 1954.

50. Woods, A. C.   Nummular keratitis and ocular brucellosis, Arch. Ophth., 35:490, 1946.

51. Zembruski, K.   Oculo-glandular form of tularemia (abstract), Am. J. Ophth., 38:448, 1954.

3

Viruses

SOME GENERAL ASPECTS OF VIRAL INFECTIONS

Viruses cause a great number of infectious diseases of man, animals, and plants. Although we will deal only with agents causing ocular diseases, certain general principles are worthy of mention.

Viruses have been known for many years, but cultivation proved difficult until 1931. In that year, Goodpasture and Woodruff developed the chick embryo technic of virus cultivation, and since then numerous viruses have been isolated. To date, more than 100 viruses are known pathogens for man.

Viruses are particles of matter, primitive yet complicated, living but unique in their mode of replication. Incapable of creating and metabolizing, they must live within cells. Hence, viral diseases are cellular diseases. The study of the virus is intimately related to cellular biochemistry. As Dr. Wendell Stanley has said,

Viruses, cancer, genes, and life are tied together. . . . Viruses can act as genes, viruses can cause cancer, and viruses are structures at the twilight zone of life partaking both of living and molecular properties.

Recently at a symposium on virus research, data were presented which concern a method of altering the heritable characteristics of viruses (e.g., by ultraviolet irradiation), thus providing further insight into the nature of the genetic "code."

Besides their individual characteristics, viruses have many common biologic properties. Most viruses may show virulence, mutation, multiplication, host range, specificity, genetic properties, and adaptation to environment. Many, except larger viruses and possibly herpes, are resistant to antibiotics and chemical therapeutic agents.

Chemical Structure of Viruses. In their simplest form, viruses consist of a nucleic acid core surrounded by a protein coat. The nucleic acid, either in the form of DNA or RNA, apparently acts as a template for further viral generation or multiplication. Plant viruses are considered to be among the simplest structures, containing only RNA, while animal viruses have DNA or RNA. Most of the known bacterial viruses (bacteriophages) contain DNA, but some recently studied have RNA. Of the animal viruses, rabbit papilloma virus has the simplest chemical structure and resembles plant viruses.

The larger viruses appear more complicated, and in addition to nucleic acid and proteins they also contain lipids and polysaccharides.

Purification and crystallization of some viruses have been accomplished.

Electron microscopy has recently elucidated some formerly invisible structural facts about viruses. The newly developed negative staining technics have revealed a great amount of information on their internal structure.

Mutation. The ability to mutate is a characteristic of all forms of life including viruses. Mutation occurs both in vivo and in tissue culture. A mutation changes the behavior of the virus and may affect its virulence, toward either enhancement or abatement. For example, the influenza virus differs in virulence every year; vaccinia virus mutates to a less virulent form than its predecessors. Epidemics may occur when a virus mutates to greater virulence and also changes its antigenic character so that the population at large is now susceptible. The range of host animals depends to some degree upon viral mutation; thus, a virus may through mutation adapt to a formerly resistant host.

Knowledge of virus mutation is an important aid to the study of heredity. Experimental mutation through the use of mutagenic agents is a way by which virus heredity may be altered.

Interference Phenomenon. When one virus modifies the infected tissue cell in such a way that another virus cannot be an invader, this is called interference phenomenon. On the other hand, dual viral infections of the same cell may occur (vaccinia and herpes simplex; measles and polio viruses). The interference phenomenon has been used only in laboratory experiments, not clinically, to prevent or decrease subsequently induced viral infection. Recently, Isaacs has described an interfering substance, which he named interferon. He defined it as a normal cell constituent, produced in excess as a defense mechanism in response to virus stimulation, especially if the viral nucleic acid is slightly changed by ultraviolet irradiation. Interferon, produced by one virus, can act against several other viruses. It is a nontoxic protein which can be isolated by conventional methods for protein purification. Isaacs feels also that cells may produce interferon in the absence of the challenging agent.

Nature and Multiplication of Viruses. Viruses are small structures, being smaller than bacteria but larger than protein molecules, and have no independent metabolism; they therefore are completely dependent upon host cells.

The virus enters a cell as an uninvited guest, demands its nutrition from the cell, and turns it into a factory to produce more viruses. Without a cell, a virus is only an inert particle. Whatever lifelike action can be ascribed to the virus begins as the virus enters the living cell. Identity remains distinct; there is no evidence that nucleic acids combine. Rather, the viruses seem to suppress the role of the cell's nucleic acid and redirect the metabolic activities toward virus synthesis. Within the cell, the viral nucleic acid acts as a template for further virus production. The newly formed virus particles emerge from infected cells and in turn affect adjacent cells, and so the cycle repeats until eventually the host cells die or production of antibodies to the viral antigens begins.

Recent work has shown that it is possible to infect cells with isolated purified viral nucleic acid. These results indicate the essential role of the nucleic acid and the secondary protective role of the protein of the viral particle.

Bacteriophage. Bacteria may act as hosts to a special group of viruses known as bacteriophages. The phage is highly host-specific. It is probable that all bacteria serve as hosts to one or more phages. There are more than 22 known staphylococcal phages. The identification of phages is rather complicated and has not yet had much practical use, since phages (except in cholera) have not been therapeutically successful. But this system is ideal to study the host-parasite relationship and mode of multiplication of viruses (biologic self-reproduction).

Growth of Viruses. Being obligate intracellular parasites, viruses grow only within living susceptible cells. They have been successfully propagated in various animals as well as in explanted tissues and cells grown in vitro. Tissue cultures and chick embryo membranes, especially chorioallantoic, are generally used culture media. During their host cells' period of active growth and metabolism, virus growth probably ceases when its required substances are exhausted.

Cultivation of viruses and the tissue culture system made possible the preparation of unlimited amounts of vaccines.

Serologic Properties and Tests. Viruses are strongly antigenic and may demonstrate one or more antigens. The ability of some viruses to stimulate antibody formation and thus create immunity is very significant. Immunity against viral infection may be short- or long-lived.

The serologic tests of agglutination, neutralization, complement fixation, and hemagglutination inhibition are used in virology. These tests are sensitive and detect viruses in very dilute solution. Unfortunately, many technical difficulties are encountered. Since viruses grow within the cells, their antigens cannot easily be separated from the involved tissue. The antigenic structure may change (mutate), and the virus can thus behave differently from one outbreak to another. Cross reaction frequently occurs with closely related viruses.

Inclusion Bodies. Inclusion bodies when present remain a significant diagnostic aid despite the development of other laboratory methods. Negri bodies of rabies and Prowazek's bodies of trachoma are virtually patho-gnomonic. Also chickenpox and smallpox, often clinically indistinguishable, may readily be diagnosed on the basis of inclusion bodies. These are cyto-plasmic in smallpox and intranuclear in chickenpox.

Morphologically, inclusion bodies represent either an aggregation of viral particles (elementary bodies) or a homogeneous mass of undetermined nature. Elementary bodies represent the infectious unit (e.g., vaccinia, tra-choma) which can be used to produce the disease experimentally.

According to their staining properties, inclusion bodies are either eosino-philic or basophilic. A single cell may contain one inclusion body or more, generally surrounded by a clear zone. The bodies may be located in the cytoplasm, within the nucleus, or both. They are usually found in epithelial cells.

The cytoplasmic inclusion bodies, chiefly belonging to the group of large viruses, are better known than those bodies residing within the nucleus. It is believed that the basophilic and eosinophilic cytoplasmic inclusion bod-ies are viral particles (elementary or initial bodies).

The intranuclear inclusion bodies are found chiefly in the small virus groups, especially the neurotropic viruses. They appear as eosinophilic homogeneous masses, and their nature is undetermined. They are not thought of as actual virus particles.

Pathology.   The pathology caused by viruses is similar to that of other infectious agents. Nevertheless there are pathologic as well as clinical char-acteristics which are pathognomonic for certain viruses. These are primarily due to their intracellular habitat.

The purulent process found in most bacterial infections is not typical for virus diseases. Necrosis and proliferation are more common features of virus pathology. Proliferation is usually produced by slow-growing mildly toxic viruses (Rous sarcoma, chickenpox, or verruca). Since the skin and mucous membranes are the main portals of entry, their epithelial cells are the first attacked. As a result, skin and mucous membrane eruptions and lesions are typical developments.

In tissues or cells grown in vitro, virus infection induces either prolifer-ative or necrotic reactions (plaque formation), and it is by these reactions that virus multiplication can be ascertained.

Viral infections call forth a typical monocytic cell response. Monocytes are macrophages which clean up tissue debris. Since the viral process is cytopathogenic, causing necrosis, cellular debris is a constant concomitant feature in viral infections. If a purulent process is present simultaneously with viral pathology, it is indicative of secondary bacterial infection. How-ever, the neutrophilic response can be due to necrotic tissue.

Classification.   There is no adequate criterion for the accurate classifi-cation of viruses. Classification on a basis of general properties divides vi-ruses into groups without particular reference to individual characteristics.

Immunologic properties are supposed to be the main criterion for classi-fication of viruses. With the present progress of serologic study, identification of individual viruses has gradually developed. There is still much confusion; further study of immunologic classification is needed.

In practice, classification by symptomatology and organ involvement is still most important for the diagnosis of viral infections. Some diseases present such typical symptomatology that they can be diagnosed clinically without further identification of the virus. On the basis of symptomatology viral diseases are distinguished as either generalized or localized.

VARIOLA, VACCINIA, AND COWPOX

These three viruses are closely related but not identical, clinically or biologically. Their origin is not clear, even today. The cowpox virus was used originally by Jenner in 1796 for vaccination against variola. Long-term laboratory propagation by various methods has altered this virus. It is be-lieved that as a result a new vaccinia virus has developed. However, some vaccinial strains probably are derived from smallpox. Differences among the three viruses are minor. All produce similar antigens and hemagglutinins which are practically identical in their reaction with immune sera. The dif-ference is in their ease of growth, host range, and, particularly, their clinical manifestation.

Variola
(Smallpox)

Variola is a highly contagious viral disease which is usually epidemic or endemic. It is primarily a skin disease with systemic involvement and has a high mortality. Since Jennerian vaccination the infection has gradually become milder and has a lower mortality.

Variola is an ancient disease well known in China, Central Africa, and India. In the Middle Ages, as a result of the Crusades, variola was widely disseminated throughout Europe and the Middle East. In Central and South America, it was introduced shortly after Columbus' first voyage. Smallpox is still a serious problem in some Asiatic countries, and infections still occur occasionally in Europe and the Americas. In the United States, several epi-demics with a high mortality occurred between 1902 and 1930 (Chapin and Smith).[2] The recurrence of epidemics or the number of sporadic cases may vary with the public laws governing vaccination. There are still some areas in the United States with no law requiring vaccination against smallpox.

Clinical Findings. After an incubation period of 10 to 13 days, the toxemia phase begins, characterized by fever and other general symptoms. A few days later, papular eruptions appear, quickly followed by the vesicular and finally the pustular stage. The lesions are distributed through the entire body but occur chiefly on the extremities and face. The eye frequently is involved. The purpuric and hemorrhagic forms of variola are very toxic and usually have a high mortality. Streptococci or other pyogenic bacteria often complicate the process and cause abscesses and pustules.

Findings in the Eye.   Primary variola of the eye is unknown, appearing only secondarily to systemic infection. The lids are often involved in the period of eruption. The lesions run the same course as elsewhere: papular, vesicular, and pustular. Severe abscess or gangrene of the lid may occur, usually in association with a bacterial infection. Variola of the lids may result in permanent scarring and consequent trichiasis and symblepharon. Keratitis and conjunctivitis frequently complicate the lid infection.

A catarrhal purulent conjunctivitis is common. In a very toxic infection, bleeding of the conjunctiva may occur, often with an associated bleeding from the nose or mouth.

Conjunctival pustules are rare; they are located typically on the bulbar conjunctiva between the limbus and the inner and outer canthus. They resemble phlyctenules but are accompanied by chemosis and severe pain.

The most serious complication of variola is corneal pustule formation. The process is usually bilateral and is often followed by perforation and sometimes by panophthalmitis. As a result, dense adherent leukoma (Plate XXV, 1) or phthisis bulbi may cause total blindness. Numbers of blind persons with pitted faces and corneal leukoma can be seen in countries where there have been epidemics of smallpox. The inner eye, particularly the uveal tract, is rarely involved. Albinotic spots of the iris as a consequence of variola have been recorded in 50 per cent of cases (Russo, 1933, in Duke-Elder, vol. 3).[3]

Laboratory Studies.   The host range is virtually restricted to man and monkeys. Animals other than monkeys have only slight susceptibility to the variola virus. As a result, the virus has not been intensively studied. However, growth of the virus on chorioallantoic membrane has been achieved (Buddingh, Lazarus).[1, 7] Whitish lesions were produced, smaller than those of vaccinia and with central necrosis. The variola virus is stable and can be propagated from dried specimens even more than one year old.

Cytoplasmic or intranuclear eosinophilic guarnieri inclusion bodies, or both, are usually found in epithelial cells from the smallpox pustule base. These bodies are large, circular or oval, homogeneous or granular, eosinophilic masses, one or more in number. Before Paschen's study, they were often regarded as protozoan in nature. In 1906 Paschen described elementary bodies which are now generally recognized as a unit of the virus. These minute bodies are always found in great numbers in the fluid from the variola and vaccinia vesicles. Paschen also concluded that the guarnieri bodies consist of viral elementary bodies. Mononuclear cells, ballooning degeneration of epithelium, and marked necrosis are additional findings. Neutrophils predominate in the pustules (Plate XXV, 4).

It is believed that virus multiplication occurs twice: first in the cells at the site of the portal of entry or within reticuloendothelial cells. From here the viruses invade the bloodstream and then spread into the skin where the second multiplication takes place.

Treatment. There is no specific therapy for variola. Convalescent serum, even in large amounts, has no effect on the infection. Prevention or treatment of bacterial complication by sulfonamides and antibiotics is important.

When ocular involvement occurs, topical therapy is added to the general treatment of the disease.

Vaccinia

Vaccinia refers to the infections caused by the virus propagated in laboratories for prophylaxis against smallpox. The origin of this virus is obscure. It is presumably cowpox virus, altered by transmission from man to man and to laboratory animals. As a result, a new entity, vaccinia virus, developed.

The main function of the vaccinia virus is to induce immunity against the smallpox virus, to which it is antigenically closely related. This suggests that some vaccinial strains have derived from the smallpox virus.

Clinical Features. The clinical manifestations of vaccinia occur following vaccination, autovaccination, or contact contamination.

The original vaccination lesion may be complicated by pyogenic organisms, with resultant cellulitis, ulceration, or severe necrosis. In the individual who has no ability to produce antibodies to the vaccinia virus, a gangrenous process may develop (Laurance et al.).[6]

Systematic reactions, such as urticarial and erythematous rashes, often result from routine vaccinations. The most severe, but fortunately rare, complications are encephalomyelitis and generalized vaccinia.

The vaccinial encephalomyelitis is similar clinically to those of variola and measles. There are several suggestions as to its origin: either from the vaccinia virus itself, allergy, or activation of another dormant neurotropic virus. Encephalomyelitis is more likely to occur if vaccination is done at a very early age—under 2 or 3 years.

Generalized vaccinia, sometimes with high mortality, may occur in persons having dermatoses of varied origin, including trauma. This also can develop merely by contact with a vaccinated person (Sommerville et al.).[13]

In a case of autovaccination the virus from the lesion of vaccination may spread to other parts of the body, including the eye. Transmission is caused by direct inoculation following scratching or rubbing the original lesions.

Findings in the Eye. Vaccinia infections of the eye may occur either by autovaccination, or more frequently, by contact contamination (Rosen).[12] The lids are most likely to become infected and pustules develop about three days after vaccination. The pustules are usually localized to the skin of the inner angulus of the lower lid (Plate XXV, 3). Occasionally a few coalescent lesions may develop. Severe swelling of the lids, preauricular and submaxillary glands, and other systemic symptoms accompany the process. Stenosis of the lacrimal passage is a rare complication of the vaccinial lesion in the inner angulus of the lower lid.

Ulcerative blepharitis is another type of vaccinial complication. The ulcers are frequently covered by gray, necrotic membranes. Purulent conjunctivitis is commonly associated with the blepharitis.

A purulent conjunctivitis without blepharitis has frequently been observed. An ulcer may occur on the lower conjunctiva. Vaccinial conjunctivitis which developed in the absence of lid lesions has been reported (Groffead and Harrison).[4]

The cornea is seldom directly infected from the original vaccinial lesion; more often, it is secondary to infection of the lid and conjunctiva. The keratitis is manifested in three forms: marginal, disciform (Perera) [11] (Plate XXV, 2), or as a corneal pustule. A pustule of the cornea is a serious condition which may result in perforation of the cornea and possibly blindness. Fortunately, the incidence is rare; it is usually associated with a corneal abrasion.

Pseudoretinitis pigmentosa with a good prognosis is recorded as an extremely rare complication of vaccination. The eye, particularly the inner part and nerve tissue, may be involved in cases of vaccinial encephalitis.

Laboratory Studies.   In contrast to variola, vaccinia virus can successfully infect many animals. Those used most extensively in the experiments are rabbits and monkeys. Rabbits in particular are highly susceptible to vaccinia, and they readily develop an acute keratitis after vaccinial inoculation of the scarified cornea. This method can therefore be used for quick diagnosis of vaccinial infection. Numerous vaccinia inclusion bodies are frequently found; they confirm the diagnosis. Vaccinia grows readily on chorioallantoic membrane. The virus may also be cultivated successfully in tissue culture, particularly of rabbit testes or kidney (van Rooyen and Rhodes).[15]

It has been adapted to grow in almost any type of tissue cells. Dermal and neural vaccinia strains have been recently developed. The effect of neural strains is best studied in monkeys.

Guarnieri variola-vaccinia eosinophilic cytoplasmic inclusion bodies consist of Paschen's elementary bodies. Inclusion bodies in vaccinia are usually cytoplasmic, while in variola they can be intranuclear as well (Plate XXV, 4). The latter are often found in cells at the base of the vesicles, while the cytoplasmic bodies are observed in cells located more superficially in the epithelial layers. These findings are quite specific in vaccinia, having been studied extensively in keratitis of rabbits. They can also be demonstrated in the epithelium of various parts of the body, e.g., skin, conjunctiva, sebaceous cysts, meibomian glands, and from the mucous membranes of the nose and throat.

Treatment.   There is no specific effective treatment. A child should be cautioned not to rub his eyes. Immune gamma globulin may be of value particularly in generalized vaccinia. For the ophthalmologist, the objective is to prevent the spread of infection from the site of inoculation. Good general hygiene of the skin should be emphasized. The usual treatment by lotion, antibiotics, or other aseptic ointment is recommended.

REFERENCES

1. Buddingh, G. J.   Infection of the chorio-allantois of the chick embryo as a diagnostic test for variola, Am. J. Hyg., 28:130, 1938.
2. Chapin, C. V., and Smith, J. J.   Permanency of mild type of smallpox, Preventive Med., 6:273, 1932.
3. Duke-Elder, W. S.   Text-book of Ophthalmology, St. Louis, Mo., C. V. Mosby Co., 1941, vol. 3, p. 2150.
4. Groffead, G. W., and Harrison, S. W.   Vaccinia conjunctivitis, Am. J. Ophth., 53:531, 1962.
5. Isaacs, A.   Interferon, Scientific American, 240:51, 1961.
6. Laurance, B., Cunliffe, A. C., and Dudgeon, J. A.   Vaccinia gangrenosa. The report of a case of prolonged generalized vaccinia, Arch. Dis. Childhood, 27:482, 1952.
7. Lazarus, A. S., Eddie, B., and Meyer, K. F.   Propagation of variola virus in the developing egg, Proc. Soc. Exper. Biol. & Med., 36:7, 1937.
8. Miller, H. G.   Acute disseminated encephalomyelitis treated with ACTH, Brit. M. J., 1:177, 1953.
9. Moffatt, A. B.   Vaccinia of the conjunctival sac, Brit. J. Ophth., 36:211, 1952.
10. Nagler, F. P. O., and Rake, G.   The use of the electron microscope in diagnosis of variola, vaccinia, and varicella, J. Bact., 55:45, 1948.
11. Perera, C. A.   Vaccinal disciform keratitis following accidental inoculation of the eyelid, Arch. Ophth., 24:352, 1940.
12. Rosen, E.   The significance of ocular complications following vaccination, Brit. J. Ophth., 33:358, 1949.
13. Sommerville, J., Napier, W., and Dick, A.   Kaposi's varicelliform eruption: record of an outbreak, Brit. J. Dermat., 63:203, 1951.
14. Stanley, W. M., and Valens, E. G.   Viruses and the Nature of Life, New York, E. P. Dutton & Co., Inc., 1961.
15. van Rooyen, C. E., and Rhodes, A. J.   Virus Diseases of Man, New York, Thos. Nelson and Sons, 1948, ch. 26-35, The variola vaccinia virus, pp. 282-429.

TRACHOMA AND INCLUSION CONJUNCTIVITIS

Both diseases are caused by large viruses of the psittacosis-lymphogranuloma group. Contrary to most others, these viruses are comparatively unstable and are sensitive to drug therapy. Large viruses are regarded as a link between typical viruses and rickettsiae. Though close to rickettsiae, large viruses differ from them in major ways: rickettsiae have arthropod vectors and do not obtain their metabolic requirements from host cells.

Members of the psittacosis-lymphogranuloma group are closely related serologically and have similar growth requirements; they all produce identical basophilic cytoplasmic inclusion bodies. However, they are clinically and epidemiologically quite different from each other, which makes their classification controversial. The association of inclusion conjunctivitis with genitourinary diseases has been established by many studies (Braley, Julianelle, Lindner, Thygeson).[5, 20, 23, 29] Inclusion conjunctivitis appears to be transmitted from the genitourinary tract. Experiments have shown that cervical scrapings may produce typical inclusion conjunctivitis, and conversely urethritis may be produced by scrapings from inclusion conjunctivitis.

Considerable difference of opinion exists as to whether trachoma and inclusion conjunctivitis are caused by identical viruses. Lindner [22] and later investigators have regarded the viruses of trachoma and "paratrachoma" (inclusion conjunctivitis) as identical. Lindner believed that two types of viruses are derived from the genitourinary tract and develop into trachoma virus as a result of passages from eye to eye. He considers inclusion conjunctivitis to be paratrachoma. This concept is not universally accepted. At present, the question of the identity of these two viruses is being considered, and new data are being presented. Jones and Collier [19] have not found any significant biologic and clinical differences between these two viruses. Mitsui [24] has observed pannus and cicatricial formation in inclusion conjunctivitis and Collier has noted the pannus. Thygeson feels that the viruses have too many clinical and epidemiologic differences to be identical.

More work is needed to prove whether they are indeed identical viruses.

Trachoma

Trachoma is a disease of the eye only, being local, without systemic involvement.

Trachoma affects millions of people in many lands and is still a major cause of blindness; antibiotics have decreased the incidence to some degree. In parts of North Africa, the Middle East, and the Orient, trachoma was once practically universal. In certain sections of the Balkans and Russia, a high incidence exists even now. Trachoma is uncommon in the United States, being localized mainly in some Indian reservations of the Southwest and among the mountain people of Kentucky, Tennessee, and New Mexico. It flourishes where poor economic conditions and poor personal hygiene prevail. Young persons and children are more susceptible to trachoma than adults, and mothers transfer the infection to their children. It is interesting that Negroes appear to be resistant to trachoma.

Clinical Features. Although great progress has been made in the laboratory study of trachoma viruses, early clinical diagnosis of trachoma is still most important.

Trachoma manifestations as well as virus strains vary in different localities. Trachoma is rare in the United States and the onset is usually acute. However, in a widespread personal experience in Russia, acute cases were rarely seen; the onset was most frequently asymptomatic. Clinical surveys have revealed numerous cases in which the patient was unaware of this infection.

Early diagnosis is difficult because there are no pathognomonic symptoms until pannus or scarring develops. Initially, trachoma is characterized by follicles which are like follicles of other origin. While not morphologically different, the fact that these follicles predominate in the upper fornix and upper tarsal conjunctiva is significant (Plate XXIII, 2). The inflammatory infiltration of the surrounding conjunctiva is a cardinal differential sign. The conjunctiva lacks its usual transparency and appears red and thick, and the individual conjunctival vessels cannot be distinguished. A deep, penetrating subepithelial and tarsal inflammatory infiltration appears. As a result of the thickened conjunctiva and tarsus, trachomatous ptosis occurs (Plate XXIII, 4).

The discharge is generally mild unless bacterial infection ensues, when it can be abundant and purulent. In Egypt, the Koch-Weeks bacillus is constantly associated with trachoma; this causes the condition to appear similar to gonococcal conjunctivitis.

Corneal involvement is most important for early diagnosis. Collier[7] and Thygeson[34] emphasize the great importance of slit lamp examination. Limbal and corneal changes are invariably present in early trachoma: vascularization of the limbus and epithelial keratitis. The slit lamp is not always available in trachomatous areas, and advanced pannus is often the presenting finding. The upper cornea is the site of pannus involvement, which may relate to the predominant infection of the upper lid (Plate XXIII, 1). Constant contact of the cornea with a rough and thickened conjunctiva is worthy of consideration in the pathogenesis of the pannus. Mechanical rubbing, direct invasion by the virus, direct absorption of toxic or allergenic substances, and disturbances of nourishment by lid pressure must be considered as contributory factors.

The finding of specific inclusion bodies helps to confirm an early tentative diagnosis. In a later stage, follicles decrease in numbers. Replacement by papillary hypertrophy and some cicatrization take place. The conjunctiva appears velvety and rough (Plate XXIII, 5). Progressive infiltration of the tissues is noted; simultaneously, the corneal process increases. According to its severity the pannus may be thin, tenuous, or very heavy (pannus crassus). The entire cornea may be involved and is a leading cause of blindness. All cases of pannus lead to corneal scarring.

The advancing margin of the pannus is often preceded by an unusually clear ulcer. Such ulcers cause corneal facets leading to decrease in vision because of changes in corneal refraction. Facets resulting from cicatrization of follicles occur at the limbus; these are so-called Herbert's pits. Bacterial infection frequently complicates the condition, with resultant severe purulent keratitis and subsequent blindness.

In later stages, various degrees of cicatrization develop (Plate XXIII, 3). The tissue infiltration and papillary hypertrophy decrease and finally disappear. A stage of pure cicatrization completes the process and results in lid deformation with trichiasis, entropion, or symblepharon. The heaviest scarring, causing incurving of the tarsus is found along the sulcus subtarsalis, an area rich in vessels. The corneal inflammation, while it may be found throughout the whole course of trachoma, usually becomes more mild or may even disappear in this stage. If in the cicatricial stage keratitis is found, it may be ascribed to the rubbing by the deformed lid.

The most tragic complication of trachoma is xerophthalmos, a type of cicatricial degeneration of the entire cornea and conjunctiva. These structures are dry, thick, and lusterless, resembling skin.

The division of trachoma into various stages is controversial. The following classification, which includes four stages, has been recommended for international use:

1. Incipient trachoma; onset of infection
2. Established trachoma
   A. Follicular hypertrophy predominant
   B. Papillary hypertrophy predominant
3. Cicatricial trachoma: appears simultaneously with remnants of inflammation
4. Healed trachoma: cicatricial

Laboratory Studies. There have been many attempts to grow the trachoma virus and finally, in 1957, T'ang[28] in China cultivated the trachoma virus in the yolk sac of embryonated eggs. This was confirmed by Collier[6] in England and Hanna et al.[15] in the United States. Since that time, cultivation of trachoma virus has been achieved in various parts of the world and confirmed by animal and volunteer inoculation (Collier et al., Dawson et al., Thygeson et al.).[7,9,33] There are described 19 or more isolated strains. The isolation of trachoma virus in tissue culture has been achieved by Gordon et al.[12] and Furness et al.[10]

The technic for isolation of the viruses is basically the same as that described by T'ang. Using conjunctival scrapings, he made three positive isolations of trachoma virus in the yolk sac of six to eight day old embryonated eggs. The material can also be taken from the conjunctiva by a swab wetted with 10 per cent broth saline. A heavy inoculum of the virus usually killed the embryos in four to eleven days. The egg-cultured virus produced a follicular conjunctivitis in rhesus monkeys and in volunteers.

Cultivation still presents difficulties. While developing the technic, it was noted that during certain seasons, the eggs were not susceptible to the trachoma virus. These were called "bad eggs," and according to Jawetz[17] the phenomenon occurs in the summer and usually lasts for one month. Variation in susceptibility was considered to be related to hormonal or nutritional disturbances among chickens. The presence of interferon can cause failure of virus growth. It is also important for virus growth to use an early passage, the fourth passage being the best (Jones).[19] Bacterial contamination, particularly by staphylococci resistant to streptomycin, has complicated some studies.

The serologic data are not complete and need further clarification. Trachoma is a process without deep invasion or systemic involvement; hence its immune response is poor. It was felt for a long time that no antibody formation or increase of host resistance occurred during active trachoma infection. Serologic studies have been accelerated by the recent advances in cultivation of the trachoma virus. There is some evidence that antibodies may affect the course of infection. Woolridge and Grayston [36] purified antigens for study in complement-fixation tests, and they detected antibodies in sera of trachomatous patients. The prevention of trachoma has been studied by many others (Grayston et al., Snyder et al.).[13, 27]

The study of inclusion bodies has a long history, but little has been added. The inclusion bodies of trachoma and inclusion conjunctivitis, known as Halberstädter-Prowazek,[14] are morphologically indistinguishable (Plate XXII, 1). They are basophilic, epithelial, and cytoplasmic, being aggregations of granules usually in the form of a cap. This appears to grasp the nucleus and may even partially occupy it. Occasionally more than one inclusion body is found in a cell. The inclusion bodies represent colonies of viruses consisting mainly of elementary bodies and a few initial bodies. The inclusion bodies are embedded in a carbohydrate matrix composed of glycogen (Thygeson).[32] The elementary bodies are infectious units which produce experimental trachoma.[30] The developmental cycle of the inclusions was established by Bedson,[2] Thygeson and others. The initial bodies develop first. Then the elementary bodies, multiplying rapidly, may occupy the entire cytoplasm. The cells rupture, liberating elementary bodies into the surrounding tissue. This is followed by the invasion of the epithelial cells. The evolution of the inclusion bodies requires about 48 hours from the time of infection.

The initial bodies are usually oval, but may vary in shape, are larger than elementary bodies, and stain dark blue. The elementary bodies are round and regular in size. They are smaller than bacteria and have often been confusingly described in the literature as red. In practice, the color is actually purplish blue (with Giemsa stain), as the designation basophilic inclusion bodies indicates. The finding of inclusion bodies is significant for early diagnosis of trachoma and for differentiation from other conjunctival processes. Their identification is not always simple, as they can be easily confused with other granules or, frequently, with pigment of varied origin, especially the melanin of dark-skinned patients. The pigment granules are distinguished by their irregular size, shape, and differing color, being green, brown, or very dark blue. They have no certain arrangement. Epithelial cells containing inclusion bodies are usually larger than normal, while those with pigment granules are of normal size (Plate XXII, 2).

In the early stage of trachoma, inclusion bodies are usually numerous and readily demonstrated in scrapings from the upper tarsal conjunctiva (Braley).[5]

Leber cells, while not specific, provide a possible clue for diagnosis (Plate XXII, 4). The author several times demonstrated Leber cells in material expressed from ripe follicles of folliculosis. These are giant histiocytic macrophages, or cells of epithelial origin, showing well-marked nucleoli. Lymphocytes and often lymphoblasts [3] and plasma cells predominate in the scraping; monocytes are also common. In the acute stage, neutrophils predominate. Vacuolized cells, the shadow cells of Humprecht, and tissue debris are additional findings in trachoma scrapings.

The pathology of trachoma is best studied in sections of tarsus with subepithelial tissue (Plate XXII, 3). Excision of the heavily involved tarsus is still an approved form of treatment. In the trachomatous area, partial or complete incision of the thickly infiltrated tarsus is the popular method of treatment. In section, heavy diffuse infiltration with lymphocytes, plasma cells, and, very rarely, follicles are found. This occurs mainly along the upper and lower arterial arches (perivascular exudation). The development of fibrous tissue in the late stage is a distinct feature.

Some observers feel that trachoma is not a single inflammatory process but a lymphoid hyperplasia.

Treatment. Copper sulfate was used as blue stone in former times, often year after year. This is now condemned, for it may create more damage than the disease itself.

Sulfonamides are considered very effective. Successful use of an immunizing vaccine has been reported recently. In the cicatricial sequel, surgical treatment is indicated. Many different operations are used. Mucous membrane grafts from the lip into the intermarginal space is an excellent approach in trichiasis. When the tarsus is heavily thickened, its partial or entire excision (Kuhnt) has had a recognized success.

If the cornea is involved, routine treatment for keratitis must be added.

Proper nutrition and personal hygiene are important in inhibiting the spread of trachoma.

Certain social conditions must be considered in the spread of trachoma. Poverty, poor nutrition, neglect of public as well as personal hygiene, and overcrowding are factors decreasing resistance and favoring dissemination of the infection.

Inclusion Conjunctivitis

Two clinical entities may be distinguished: inclusion conjunctivitis of the newborn and inclusion conjunctivitis of adults.

Inclusion Conjunctivitis of Newborn (Ophthalmia Neonatorum, Inclusion Blennorrhea). Instead of the confusing term blennorrhea, we prefer to use inclusion conjunctivitis, as proposed by Thygeson.

This is an acute, purulent conjunctivitis occurring five to ten days after birth. As the infant passes through the birth canal, it is infected with the virus. The process is characterized by a profuse purulent exudate (Plate XXIV, 1). It may begin bilaterally or unilaterally, in which case the second eye is involved three to seven days later. The lower lid is more severely involved than the upper. Papillary hypertrophy is not uncommon; in severe cases, pseudomembrane formation can be seen. The process is self-limited, with complete healing in ten to twelve days. Chronic cases are extremely rare, almost unknown. The cornea is uninvolved. Eye-to-eye contamination is very rare; the infection is commonly limited to a single member of the family.

The disease must be differentiated from gonococcal conjunctivitis of the newborn. The short incubation period, two to three days, and the laboratory finding of gonococci are important for diagnosis.

Inclusion Conjunctivitis of Adults (Swimming Pool Conjunctivitis). This is an acute follicular conjunctivitis. The disease is caused by the same virus as is inclusion blennorrhea but has several different clinical features. The discharge is scanty in adults. There is more roughness and redness of the conjunctiva, with follicles and papillary formation (Plate XXIV, 2); the preauricular nodes are enlarged (in the newborn this is absent). The process is usually unilateral, of long duration, sometimes lasting years, and mildly contagious. Poorly chlorinated swimming pools, infected by viruses from the genitourinary tract, are sources of infection. It is differentiated from trachoma on the basis of lack of scarring and absence of corneal involvement, and eye-to-eye contamination is almost unknown.

Typical inclusion bodies differentiate this condition from other forms of follicular conjunctivitis.

Laboratory Studies. This question has been discussed in the section on trachoma. Numerous investigators have previously studied the virus, especially significant contributions having been made by Allen, Braley, Julianelle, Thygeson, and others.[1, 4, 21, 29]

However, attempts to cultivate inclusion blennorrhea viruses failed. Only in 1959 the first isolation of the virus was reported by Jones, Collier, and Smith.[18] They employed the same technic as had been used for isolation of the trachoma virus, in yolks of embryonated eggs. Two isolations of the virus were made: one from inclusion conjunctivitis, the other from the cervix. Jones and Collier later established that a virus strain present in the female genital tract, isolated from the resultant neonatal blennorrhea, is capable of producing trachoma in the adult eye. The first isolation in the United States of the inclusion blennorrhea virus was reported in 1960 by Hanna et al.[16] Later, its successful growth in cell culture was reported.[8, 11] Recently Thygeson et al.[35] achieved positive inoculation of human volunteers with egg-grown inclusion conjunctivitis virus.

Laboratory studies have demonstrated marked similarity between the viruses of inclusion conjunctivitis and trachoma. In cultivation technic, serology, and immunology these viruses are alike (see page 107). Although closely related biologically their clinical manifestations and epidemiology are different.

Isolation of the virus and purification and concentration technics in the yolks of embryonated eggs greatly accelerated studies of its serology and immunity.

Cytologic features are the same in the scrapings from both clinical entities of inclusion conjunctivitis. Inclusion bodies, indistinguishable from those of trachoma, are most significant for diagnosis. Contrary to trachoma, they are usually found in scrapings from the lower lid. Predominant neutrophilic and monocytic responses are additional differential characteristics. Monocytes are usually markedly vacuolized (Plate XXIV, 3).

Treatment. Treatment is not a problem in the newborn, as the condition is self-limited. The process responds readily to local treatment with sulfonamides; additionally, aureomycin or Terramycin may be effective. In adults, local treatment with the above-mentioned drugs, plus systemic treatment if the condition does not respond, may be needed to prevent a chronic course.

REFERENCES

1. Allen, J. H.   Inclusion blennorrhea, Am. J. Ophth., 27:833, 1944.
2. Bedson, S. P.   Observation on the developmental forms of psittacosis virus, Brit. J. Exper. Path., 14:267, 1933.
3. Biantovskaya (Fedukowicz), E. T., and Shapiro, E. I.   Diagnostic significance of cytologic examination of follicles of adenoid tissue in trachoma, Sovet. vestnik. oftal., 4:596, 1934.
4. Braley, A. E.   Inclusion blennorrhea. A study of the pathologic changes in the conjunctiva and cervix, Am. J. Ophth., 21:1203, 1938.
5. ———   The relation between the virus of trachoma and the virus of inclusion blennorrhea, Arch. Ophth., 22:393, 1939.
6. Collier, L. H., and Sowa, J.   Isolation of trachoma virus in embryonate eggs, Lancet, 1:993, 1958.
7. ———   Duke-Elder, W. S., and Jones, B. R.   Experimental trachoma produced by cultured virus, Brit. J. Ophth., 42:705, 1958.
8. ———   Growth characteristics of inclusion blennorrhea virus in cell cultures, Ann. New York Acad. Sc., 98:42, 1962.
9. Dawson, C. R., Mordhorst, C. H., and Thygeson, P.   Infection of rhesus and cynomolgus monkeys with egg-grown viruses of trachoma and inclusion conjunctivitis, Ann. New York Acad. Sc., 98:167, 1962.
10. Furness, G., Graham, D., Reeve, P., and Collier, L. H.   The growth of trachoma and inclusion blennorrhea viruses in cell culture, Rev. Internat. Trachoma, 4:574, 1960.
11. ———   Graham, D. M., and Reeve, P.   The titration of trachoma and inclusion blennorrhoea viruses in cell cultures, J. Gen. Microbiol., 23:613, 1960.
12. Gordon, F. B., Quan, A. L., and Trimmer, R. W.   Morphological observation on trachoma virus in cell culture, Science, 131:733, 1960.

13. Grayston, J. T., Wang, S., Woolridge, R. L., Yang, Y., and Johnston, P. B. Trachoma-studies of etiology, laboratory diagnosis, and prevention, J.A.M.A., 172: 1577, 1960.

14. Halberstädter, L., and Prowazek, S. Ueber Chlamydozoen befunde bei Blennorrhöe neonatorum non gonorrhoica, Berlin, Klin. Wchnschr., 46:1839, 1909.

15. Hanna, L., Jawetz, E., Thygeson, P., and Dawson, C. Trachoma viruses isolated in United States. I. Growth in embryonated eggs, Proc. Soc. Exper. Biol. & Med., 104:142, 1960.

16. ———— Zichosch, J., Jawetz, E., Vaughan, D. G., Jr., and Thygeson, P. Virus isolated from inclusion conjunctivitis of newborn (inclusion blennorrhea), Science, 132:1660, 1960.

17. Jawetz, E. Seasonal insusceptibility of embryonated eggs to viruses of trachoma and inclusion conjunctivitis, Ann. New York Acad. Sc., 98:31, 1962.

18. Jones, B. R., Collier, L. H., and Smith, C. H. Isolation of virus from inclusion blennorrhea, Lancet, 1:902, 1959.

19. ———— and Collier, L. H. Inoculation of man with inclusion blennorrhea virus, Ann. New York Acad. Sc., 98:212, 1962.

20. Julianelle, L. A. Relation of inclusion blennorrhea to swimming-bath conjunctivitis as determined by an accidental transmission, Proc. Soc. Exper. Biol. & Med., 36:617, 1937.

21. ———— and Harrison, R. W. Studies on inclusion blennorrhea, Am. J. Ophth., 21:1230, 1938.

22. Lindner, K. Infektions versuche von Trachom mit Paratrachom des Neugeborenen (Einschlussblennorrhöe), Arch. Ophth., 133:479, 1935.

23. ———— Gonoblennorrhöe, Einschlussblennorrhöe und Trachom, Graef's Arch. Ophth., 78:245, 1911.

24. Mitsui, Y. Etiology of trachoma, Am. J. Ophth., 32:1189, 1949.

25. ———— and Suzuki, A. Electron microscopy of trachoma virus in section, Arch. Ophth., 56:429, 1956.

26. Mohsenine, H., and Darougar, S. The provocative effect of cortisone on trachoma, Rev. Internat. Trachoma, 34:336, 1957.

27. Snyder, J. C., Bell, S. D., Jr., and Murray, E. S. Attempt to immunize a volunteer (with formalin-inactivated virus) against experimental trachoma induced by Saudi Arabian strain, Ann. New York Acad. Sc., 98:368, 1962.

28. T'ang, F. F., Chang, H. L., Huang, Y. T., and Wang, K. C. Studies on the etiology of trachoma with special reference to isolation of the virus in chick embryo, Chinese M. J., 75:429, 1957.

29. Thygeson, P. The etiology of inclusion blennorrhea, Am. J. Ophth., 17:1019, 1934.

30. ———— Proctor, F. I., and Richards, P. The etiologic significance of the elementary body in trachoma, Am. J. Ophth., 18:811, 1935.

31. ———— and Mengert, W. F. The virus of inclusion conjunctivitis, Arch. Ophth., 15:377, 1936.

32. ———— The matrix of the epithelial cell inclusion of trachoma, Am. J. Path., 14:455, 1938.

33. ———— and Crocker, T. T. Observations on experimental trachoma and inclusion conjunctivitis, Am. J. Ophth., 42:76, 1956.

34. ———— The limbus and cornea in experimental and natural human trachoma and inclusion conjunctivitis, Ann. New York Acad. Sc., 98:201, 1962.

35. ———— Hanna, L., Dawson, C., Zichosch, J., and Jawetz, E. Inoculation of human volunteer with egg-grown inclusion conjunctivitis virus, Am. J. Ophth., 53:786, 1962.

36. Woolridge, R. L., and Grayston, J. T. Further studies with a complement fixation test for trachoma, Ann. New York Acad. Sc., 98:314, 1962.

HERPES SIMPLEX

Manifestations of herpes simplex virus infection are frequent and varied. There are several clinical entities, characterized by vesicular eruption of the skin and mucous membranes; these variations are due to virulence of the strain, degree of local immunity, and history of previous attack. Herpes simplex virus commonly infects the eye, having a special predilection for the cornea.

In the United States, herpetic keratitis is a troublesome, often chronic disease and the most common cause of blindness. Its incidence and severity appear to be increasing. Thygeson et al.[19] and Kimura et al.[13] feel the increasing frequency coincides with recent wars and the antibiotic and steroid eras.

Clinical Features. Herpes simplex is divided clinically into primary herpes and recurrent herpes.

Primary Herpes Simplex. Initial or primary herpes simplex usually occurs in children aged six months to 5 years; it is rare in adulthood. Infants appear to be born with maternal herpes-specific antibodies which disappear within six months. From then to 24 months, sensitivity to herpes infection is greatest. Gingivostomatitis, vulvovaginitis, Kaposi's eruption, and acute keratoconjunctivitis[8] are common primary herpes manifestations. These are usually accompanied by systemic involvement, fever, and enlargement of regional glands. The infection can be severe, even fatal. Nevertheless, about 90 per cent of primary herpes cases are asymptomatic.

Severe infection may occur in premature infants, and a fatal viremia may result. The mechanism is not known; possibly there is a low titer of maternal antibodies, a high dose of the virus, or according to Rake,[16] greater vulnerability of premature cells. The disease may be associated with herpes of the maternal genitalia.

After the first attack, antibodies against the herpes virus are demonstrated. This was confirmed when Buddingh et al.[4] reported the presence of neutralizing antibodies in 90 per cent of healthy persons over the age of 15. The finding of specific antibodies is regarded as evidence of previous primary herpes infection. It is also recognized that primary herpes gives rise to a latent infection which may persist throughout life. This may be activated by many unspecific stimuli and becomes recurrent.

Recurrent Herpes Simplex. Common factors appearing to reactivate the latent herpes virus are: various fevers—pneumonia, malaria, or others—emotional disturbances, physical trauma such as cold or heat, chemical factors, and others. The exact mechanism of activation is unknown. The evidence of recurrent infection is the presence of specific antibodies in convalescent serum (Andrewes and Carmichael).[1] During the primary attack, antibodies are absent. They appear about 10 days after onset. The recurrent process is usually localized and without systemic involvement. The commonest clinical entities are: herpes febriles, herpes labialis, herpes genitalis, and herpes of the cornea.

If chronic eczema is present, herpes virus infection causes a severe condition called eczema herpeticum.

Findings in the Eye. Herpes simplex virus has a primary affinity for the cornea, causing a dendritic keratitis which is pathognomonic.

Primary herpetic dendritic keratitis occurs rarely, and seldom before six months of age. However, it has been recognized in premature infants. In infancy and childhood, the process is usually bilateral and more severe than in adults (Plate XXVII, 1, 2). It is accompanied by systemic manifestations, enlargement of regional nodes, or occasionally by central nervous system involvement.

Superficial (epithelialis) punctate or diffuse keratitis has also been considered a primary manifestation of herpes simplex. The same clinical picture can be found in other conditions, particularly epidemic keratoconjunctivitis. Therefore, laboratory diagnosis is necessary. However, loss of corneal sensitivity may distinguish herpetic keratitis from epidemic keratoconjunctivitis.

An acute follicular conjunctivitis is usually found with primary herpetic keratitis in children, but adults' primary herpetic keratitis is generally associated with an acute ulcerative blepharitis.

In recurrent herpes, dendritic keratitis is the commonest ocular sign. This condition occurs unilaterally, predominantly in adult males (Plate XXVII, 5). Regional lymph nodes are uninvolved, and there is no systemic symptomatology. The keratitis evolves as a superficial punctate form with erosions; within 24 hours a small dendritic ulcer may develop. Vesicles in groups or rows may appear prior to ulceration; they rupture promptly and often escape detection. The branches of the dendritic figure have knobby extremities.

The process is usually chronic and recurrent, points not well explained. A possible explanation appears to have been overlooked. The virus can be neurotropic and usually affects the central cornea, which is richest in nerve branches. As a result, the keratitis is primarily neurotrophic, as evidenced by loss of sensitivity. It is known that neurotrophic keratitis of any origin presents a problem to ophthalmologists. Dendritic keratitis, even mild, is usually followed by scarring. However, it may be complicated by secondary bacterial or fungus infection which may result from steroid therapy. Steroid therapy, particularly in the early stages of a herpetic keratitis, is quite dangerous. Thygeson pointed out that hypopyon keratitis may present a diagnostic problem if a preceding dendritic keratitis has not been observed. Total corneal anesthesia and an indolent process are clues to prior herpes infection.

Besides dendritic keratitis there are a variety of herpetic keratitides, both superficial and interstitial. Among the superficial types are: punctate, marginal, striatum, stellatum, band-shaped, and filamentous. The filamentous form develops perhaps as a result of prolonged edema or too frequent cauterization. The function of the lacrimal glands is usually normal. The herpetic keratitides are often confused with similar conditions of other etiology. Braley [3] pointed out that superficial punctate keratitis may often be mistaken for epidemic keratoconjunctivitis. Among the deep herpetic keratitides, disciform is most frequent (Plate XXVII, 4). Thygeson and Kimura [21] regard disciform keratitis as principally caused by herpes simplex and only rarely caused by herpes zoster, vaccinia, mumps, or varicella. Benign and severe disciform types of herpetic keratitis occur. In the latter, necrosis and perforation are seen. The increasing number of severe cases recently reported may follow steroid therapy. Several authors indicate that disciform keratitis may be associated with hypersensitivity or frequent use of iodine cauterization.

Herpetic conjunctivitis, common in children, is rarely seen in adults. It is either a follicular or, less frequently, a membranous type; neither is distinguishable from similar manifestations of other origin. Prior or simultaneous appearance of vesicular skin eruptions is diagnostically important. Vesicles are occasionally seen on the palpebral conjunctiva. These promptly break down, leaving superficial ulcers.

Acute herpetic blepharitis may be found in adults, being characterized by formation of vesicles along the cilial lines; the vesicles break down and ulcerate. The ulcers are covered by glistening grayish membranes which have a tendency to spread over the palpebral conjunctiva. The lid margins become edematous and a concurrent dermatitis of the upper lid is often present. Some of our cases also showed marked enlargement of the preauricular glands (oculoglandular Parinaud's syndrome).

Recurrent indolent herpetic iritis and iridocyclitis of a hemorrhagic type are recorded. They often result in secondary glaucoma. These are usually preceded by severe disciform keratitis.

A case of recurrent sympathetic ophthalmia due to herpes has been described.[5]

METAHERPES.   The term metaherpes refers to the keratitis which develops on the site of a healed dendritic keratitis. This appears in various forms, mainly as superficial round or oval ulcers, often with scalloped borders, but not in a dendritic form. Superficial infiltrates or a deep interstitial process may be seen. Metaherpes develops slowly, and contrary to the condition in dendritic keratitis, epithelial cells are firmly fixed. The process does not heal readily, and its etiology is unknown. Other viruses or bacteria are suggested causative agents. In some cases it can be an allergic manifestation. Since metaherpes occurs in the area of anesthesia, the keratitis is possibly neuroparalytic. Hogan regards the name metaherpes as confusing. He would prefer to designate the process "chronic post-herpetic corneal ulceration."

Laboratory Studies. Current development in laboratory diagnosis is given in an excellent review by Howard and Kaufman.[11]

The herpes virus is dermatotropic, but virulent strains may become neurotropic. Herpes simplex has a wide range of susceptible hosts. It grows readily on the chorioallantoic membrane of 10 to 13 day old embryonated eggs,[17] producing pocks containing Lipschütz inclusion bodies. Herpes virus can also be propagated in tissue culture;[7] chick embryo or rabbit kidney tissue is considered best. Hanna et al.[9] have shown the advantage of HeLa cell culture in detecting both herpes simplex and adenovirus.

Rabbit cornea has been widely used experimentally because of its marked susceptibility to herpes simplex. Viral inoculation of the scarified cornea causes severe keratitis within 24 hours. Propagation of the virus can be achieved by passages. Rabbits are now used less because of the advantages of new technics, such as tissue culture technics. The fact that the herpes virus has been isolated from healthy carriers must be considered in establishing its etiologic role.

The method of collecting specimens is important. Swabbed or scraped material must be collected in the acute stage. Culture medium 199 is the most suitable for preserving specimens. This can serve as inoculum for embryonated eggs, animals, and tissue culture. The use of saline is not recommended; it may inhibit the growth of herpes. The specimen should be studied as early as possible, but if necessary it can be stored for a short time in the freezer compartment of the refrigerator.

Cytologic study is based on scrapings and sections. For the scrapings, Giemsa stain is commonly used. One finds homogeneous intranuclear eosinophilic masses described by Lipschütz as herpes simplex inclusion bodies. These are now regarded as the end stage of a two-stage virus development. In the first stage, the inclusion bodies appear as a basophilic Feulgen-positive substance (DNA) consisting of viral particles. In the second stage these particles gradually disappear and are replaced by a nonviral Feulgen-negative eosinophilic mass (Lipschütz bodies) thought to be a product of cellular degeneration caused by the virus. It has also been referred to as a nuclear scar. Lipschütz bodies are easily demonstrated experimentally, but rarely, and usually in an early stage in human herpes. Giant cells containing 2 to 15 or more nuclei are regarded as significant for herpes simplex. Consistent demonstration of these cells in corneal or skin scrapings may justify the diagnosis. A special method for staining the scrapings is described by Lennette.[14] Ballooning degeneration of epithelial cells as a result of fluid collection may be a diagnostic aid. Polynuclear cells are often found in association with secondary bacterial infection. Cytologic examination has some value, especially in association with other diagnostic data (Plate XXVII, 3).

The question of immunity is in doubt, as recurrent herpes is very frequent. However, it has been demonstrated that recurrent lesions do not commonly appear on the same site. If they do occur, the infection is shorter and milder. Also, a number of specific antibodies have been found in convalescent sera. Coons and others reported fluorescein-labeled antibodies.[6] There are many theories on recurrence of herpes: 1, the antibody titer is probably low; 2, antibodies are not completely specific; 3, some viruses have a very high virulence; 4, immunity is confined to the area of the healed lesions. At present no satisfactory explanation is available.

Treatment. Numerous remedies have been advocated for treatment of dendritic keratitis. The reader is referred to a comprehensive discussion by Thomas.[18] Iodine therapy is a popular method. Its purpose is to destroy the epithelial cells harboring the viruses. Therefore the corneal epithelial cells of the involved and adjacent areas, sometimes of the entire cornea, have to be removed. The epithelial cells are loosely connected with the cornea and therefore easily denuded. First, anesthetize the cornea; then use a fine applicator wetted with tincture of iodine. Cauterization must be done thoroughly to obtain a good result. After cauterization, repeated instillation of 4 per cent cocaine hydrochloride is recommended by Thomas. This precipitates iodides, with a resultant dark brown color of the area. Epithelial cells are quickly regenerated, and healing usually follows without scarring. Atropine drops and light bandaging complete the procedure.

The question of steroid therapy in dendritic keratitis is controversial. Its use is condemned, especially in the acute stage. However, in disciform keratitis where hypersensitivity is suggested, steroids may have a place.

Surgical treatments such as lamellar grafting have recently received attention (Hogan).[10]

Gamma globulin, administered topically and parenterally, has not been particularly useful. Antibiotics are used chiefly for secondary bacterial infections; they have no recognized specific effect on any type of herpes simplex. However, very encouraging results have been recorded concerning IDU (5-iodo-2'-deoxyuridine).

The viral antibiotic, IDU, was first used experimentally by Kaufman.[12] Clinical observations are not yet sufficient to prove fully its therapeutic effects, although there is a possibility that it may cure herpetic keratitis even when it is far advanced. Unfortunately, even after successful treatment, recurrence frequently takes place.

REFERENCES

1. Andrewes, C. H., and Carmichael, E. A.   A note on the presence of antibodies to herpes virus in post-encephalitic and other human sera, Lancet, 1:857, 1930.
2. Braley, A. E.   Experimental herpes simplex, Am. J. Ophth., 35:1737, 1952.
3. ———   Acute herpetic keratoconjunctivitis, Am. J. Ophth., 43(Part 2):105, 1957.
4. Buddingh, G. J., Schrum, D. I., Lanier, J. C., and Guidry, D. J.   Studies of the natural history of herpes simplex infections, Pediatrics, 11:595, 1953.

Plates XXII–XXIX

PLATE XXII

1. Cytology of trachoma in scraping (Giemsa stain). Note basophilic cytoplasmic inclusion bodies (Prowazek) in epithelial cells (see page 117). Lymphocytes and plasma cells are typically found in trachoma.

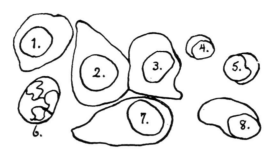

1. ⎱
2. ⎰ Basophilic cytoplasmic inclusion
3. ⎱ bodies (Prowazek) in epithelial
7. ⎰ cells

4. ⎱ Lymphocytes
5. ⎰
6. Neutrophil
8. Plasma cell

2. Cytoplasmic granules. These are not to be confused with trachomatous inclusion bodies (see page 117).

3. Pathology of trachoma in section (hematoxylin-eosin stain). Follicles are shown, each consisting of a peripheral zone of lymphocytes and a germinal center of large lymphoblasts, monocytes, and epithelioid cells. Note round cell infiltration of stroma. On the right, a hypertrophic papilla with beginning fibrosis (red streaks) is shown.

4. Leber cell. The Leber cell is a giant macrophage, significant but not specific for trachoma. Its cytoplasmic border is ill-defined. The cytoplasm engulfs debris from distintegrating cells (nuclear material is dark, cytoplasmic is light).

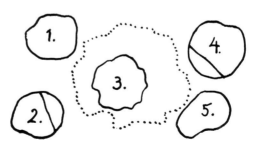

1. ⎱
2. ⎰ Degenerated lymphocytes   3.   Leber cell
4. ⎱
5. ⎰

PLATE XXII   129

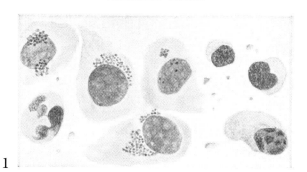

1

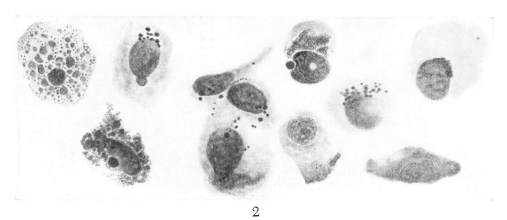

2

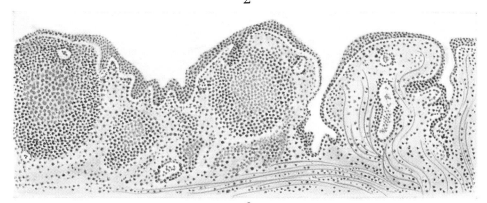

3

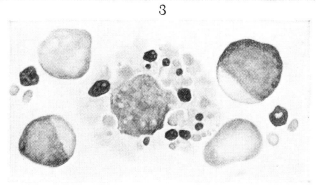

4

PLATE XXIII

1. Pannus trachomatosus. Diffuse vascular keratitis. Typically, the superficial branching vessels invade the upper limbus and run subepithelially in the cornea. Note the diffuse opacity and two isolated infiltrates.

2. Trachomatous follicular conjunctivitis in the early stage of trachoma. The follicles are indistinguishable from those in other follicular conjunctivitis or folliculosis (see page 115). Localization on upper tarsal conjunctiva, with infiltration of surrounding tissue, is significant for differential diagnosis of early trachoma.

3. Scarring of upper tarsal conjunctiva in trachoma. The scar is usually horizontal, particularly along the sulcus subtarsalis; entropion often results.

4. Trachomatous ptosis. The upper lid droops due to the weight of the infiltrated lid or from infiltration of the levator muscle at the site of its insertion.

5. Trachoma in later stage. The entire upper tarsal conjunctiva is covered by hypertrophic papillae (red, rough, irregular in size, flat on top, and hard). The whitish line between papillae indicates scarring.

PLATE XXIII 131

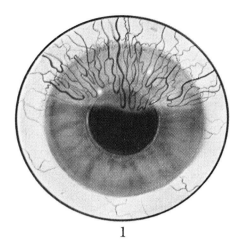

1

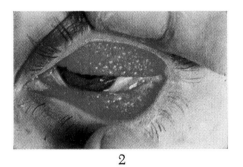

2

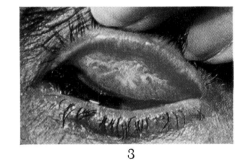

3

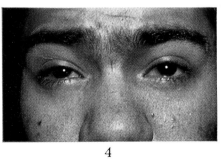

4

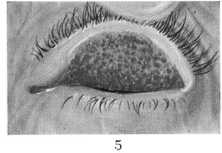

5

PLATE XXIV

1. Inclusion conjunctivitis of newborn (ophthalmia neonatorum). Acute purulent conjunctivitis occurring 5 to 10 days after birth. Conjunctiva of lower lid is
predominantly involved; take the scraping from the lower conjunctiva. The process is usually mild. In severe cases pseudomembranes occur. The cornea is uninvolved. Cytoplasmic basophilic inclusion bodies (illustrated in 3, below) confirm
the diagnosis.

2. Inclusion conjunctivitis of adults (swimming pool conjunctivitis). The unilateral process begins as an acute bacterial conjunctivitis (moderate secretion).
Follicles later appear, possibly on both conjunctivae, and papillary hypertrophy
may develop. There is no scarring or corneal involvement. Cytoplasmic basophilic
inclusion bodies (illustrated in 3, below) are found.

3. Scraping (Giemsa stain) from inclusion conjunctivitis. Cytoplasmic basophilic
inclusion bodies in epithelial cells are indistinguishable from those in trachoma
(see page 117). In the typical cell response, neutrophils and monocytes are seen.
Monocytes are usually vacuolized. Giant multinucleated cells may be found.

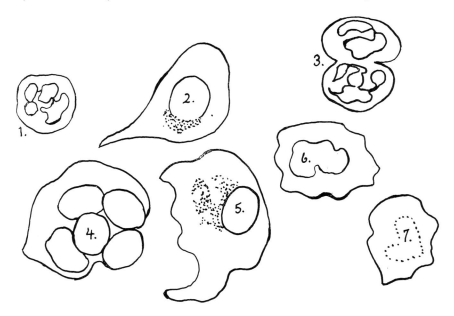

1. ⎱
3. ⎰ Neutrophils

2. ⎱ Epithelial cells with Prowazek's
5. ⎰ inclusion bodies

4. Multinucleated cell

6. ⎱ Monocytes with vacuolization
7. ⎰ and autolysis

PLATE XXIV   133

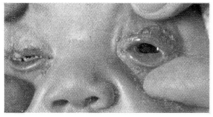

1

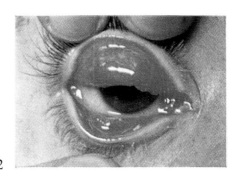

2

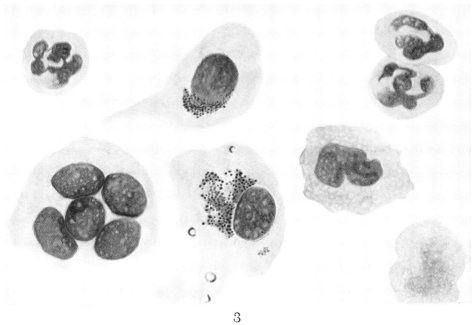

3

PLATE XXV

1. Sequelae of corneal variola pustule. Anterior staphyloma, with resulting permanent blindness. Note pox marks on skin.

2. Vaccinial disciform keratitis (similar to other disciform keratitis). A type of avascular interstitial keratitis. The opacity is not dense. The process is benign. Grayish lines near the disc are Descemet's folds.

3. Vaccinia of lid. Typical transmission to lid (inner angulus usual) from the site of vaccination, showing on arm.

4. Guarnieri variola-vaccinia inclusion bodies (Giemsa stain). Inclusions are eosinophilic, cytoplasmic (in variola, intranuclear as well), consisting of Paschen's elementary bodies. Guarnieri bodies are rarely found except in experimental studies. Ballooning degeneration, monocytes, and neutrophils are additional cytologic characteristics.

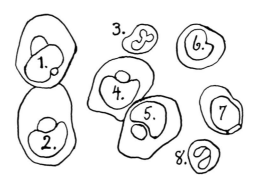

1.
2. Cytoplasmic eosinophilic
4. Lipschütz inclusion bodies
5.

6.   Monocyte

3.
8. Neutrophils

7.   Ballooning degeneration

PLATE XXV   135

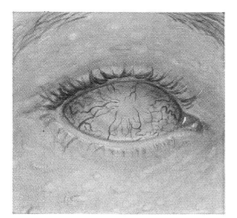

1

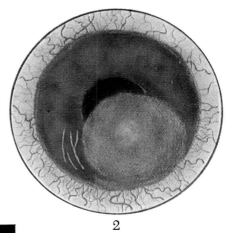

2

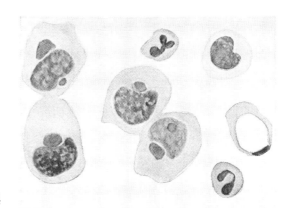

3

4

PLATE XXVI

1. Zoster (herpes zoster, shingles, zona). Severe ulcerative necrotic process distributed along supraorbital branch. Usually unilateral (except in syphilis).

2. Disciform keratitis (usual type). The corneal disc-shaped opacity in the interstitial tissue is not dense; its surface may be eroded. Descemet's folds sometimes occur.

3. Superficial keratitis. Mainly punctate. Also note the vesicles in groups and rows. These rupture promptly and are rarely seen. (Both types, in 2 and 3, can occur in zoster.)

4. Cytology in scraping (Giemsa stain). Eosinophilic, intranuclear Lipschütz inclusion bodies (similar to those in herpes simplex) are pictured. Ballooning degeneration and multinucleated giant cells are additional findings.

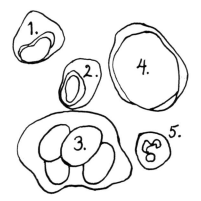

1.) Eosinophilic intranuclear	3. Multinucleated giant cell
2.) Lipschütz inclusion bodies	
5. Neutrophil	4. Ballooning degeneration

5. Varicella. Although a disease of childhood, varicella virus may become latent and manifest as a zoster in adulthood.

PLATE XXVI   137

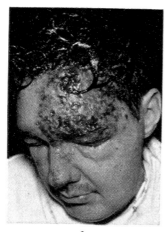

1

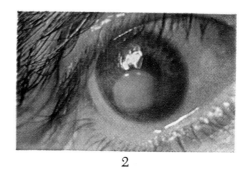

2

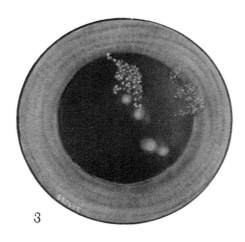

3

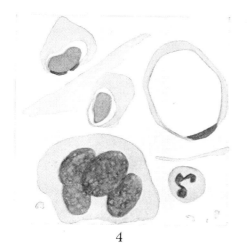

4

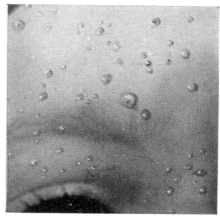

5

PLATE XXVII

1 and 2. Primary bilateral dendritic corneal ulcers in newborn baby. This condition is rare, usually bilateral, and accompanied by systemic manifestations. Dendritic shape and loss of sensitivity indicate herpetic origin.

3. Cytology in scraping (Giemsa stain). Eosinophilic intranuclear Lipschütz inclusion bodies similar to zoster. Giant multinucleated cell, usually found in herpes simplex. Monocytes and neutrophils are commonly found.

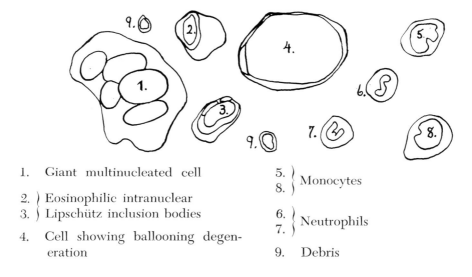

1. Giant multinucleated cell	5. | Monocytes 8. /
2.) Eosinophilic intranuclear 3. } Lipschütz inclusion bodies	6. | Neutrophils 7. /
4. Cell showing ballooning degeneration	9. Debris

4. Disciform keratitis (late stage). Dense, deep opacity invaded by deep vessels; scarring results.

5. Recurrent dendritic corneal ulcer (in adult). Commonly chronic, unilateral, and recurrent. Branching figure and loss of corneal sensitivity are regarded as pathognomonic for herpes simplex. No systemic manifestations.

PLATE XXVII 139

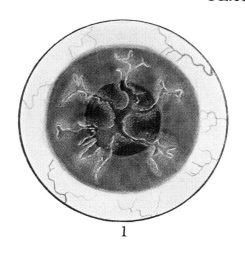

1

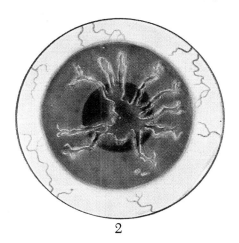

2

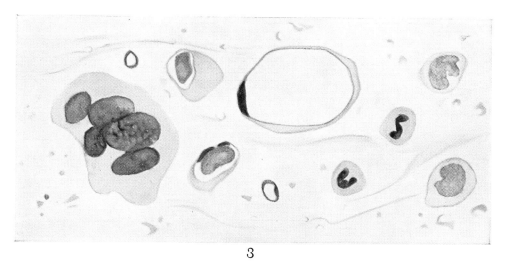

3

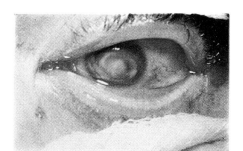

4

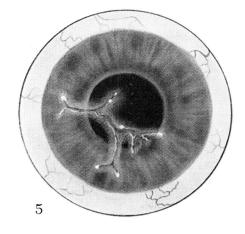

5

PLATE XXVIII

1. Acute herpetic blepharitis. Several broken vesicles are present on the margin and skin of the lids. The lids are markedly swollen. Preauricular glands are enlarged.

2. Acute follicular conjunctivitis (same patient as 1). Lower conjunctiva is involved. Bulbar conjunctiva is intensively hyperemic. Note unusual, markedly circumscribed swelling.

3. Acute herpetic blepharoconjunctivitis. Along the cilial line broken vesicles have resulted in an ulcerated area which, unlike usual blepharitis, is covered by a grayish membrane. Follicular conjunctivitis, mainly in the lower fornix, developed two days after onset. Enlargement of preauricular and submaxillary glands (oculoglandular Parinaud's syndrome). Herpes simplex virus isolated on Hela cell tissue culture.

4. Follicular conjunctivitis associated with mild sore throat and fever (pharyngoconjunctival fever). Large follicles are localized mainly in the lower fornix. Enlargement of preauricular and, particularly, submaxillary glands. Adenovirus Type 3 was isolated.

5. Epidemic keratoconjunctivitis (EKC). Subepithelial, small, grayish, irregular, multiple lesions. Localization in central (pupillary) area is typical for EKC. The disease was evidently caused by adenovirus Type 8.

6. Cytology in scraping (Giemsa stain). Mononuclear cells: monocytes and lymphocytes predominate. Large epithelial cells may be found. Similar cytology is found in other viral conjunctivitides.

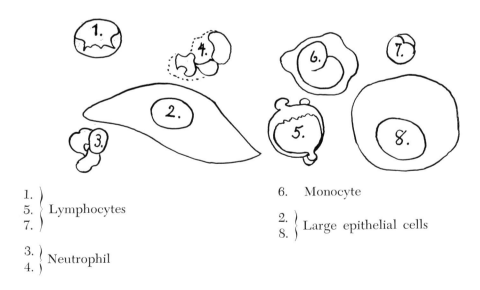

1.
5. } Lymphocytes
7.

3.
4. } Neutrophil

6.   Monocyte

2.
8. } Large epithelial cells

PLATE XXVIII

141

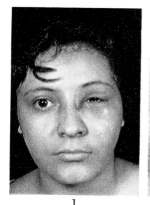

1

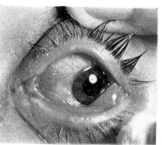

2

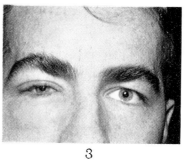

3

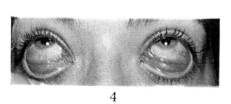

4

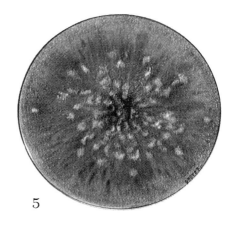

5

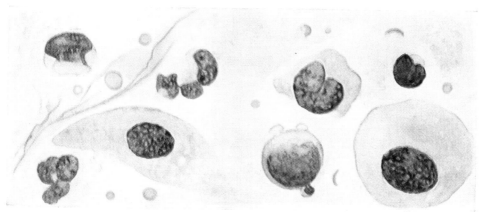

6

PLATE XXIX

1. Molluscum contagiosum of lids. Uninflamed, round, waxy, white lesions. The summit is usually umbilicated and has a tiny black spot. If the lesion is situated at the lid margin, the cornea and conjunctiva can be involved.

2. Pannus (develops if molluscum contagiosum is situated at the lid margin). This is localized (similarly to trachoma) at the upper part of the cornea. Probably toxic, it heals after removal of lid lesion. The process may be associated with follicular conjunctivitis.

3. Inclusion bodies of molluscum contagiosum (in section, stained with hematoxylin-eosin). Henderson-Paterson cytoplasmic eosinophilic inclusion bodies. These are composed of elementary bodies aggregated in globular masses (separated by septa) which press the shrunken nucleus (shown by dark staining) to the cell wall.

4. Cornu cutaneum (cutaneous horn). A rare lesion consisting of horny epithelium; regarded as horn wart, probably viral.

5. Wart (verruca filiformis). Epidermal and papillary growths of viral origin; soft and flexible, typically situated on face, neck, and eyelids. Multiple lesions are disseminated in the bearded area by shaving. Involvement of the cornea and conjunctiva (as in molluscum contagiosum) may occur if the lesion is situated at the lid margin.

PLATE XXIX   143

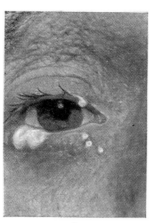

1

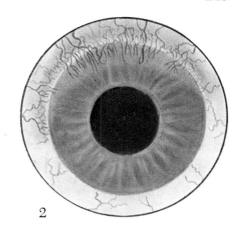

2

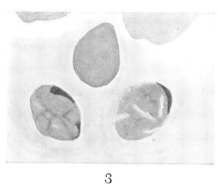

3

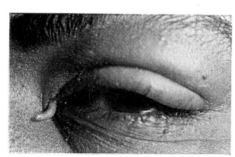

4

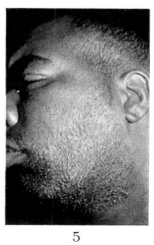

5

5. Cavara, V., and Di Ferdinando, R. Sympathetic ophthalmia and herpetic infection (abstract), Am. J. Ophth., 32:1313, 1949.

6. Coons, A. H., Creech, H. J., and Jones, R. N. Immunological properties of antibody containing a fluorescent group, Proc. Soc. Exper. Biol. & Med., 47:200, 1941.

7. Doane, F., Rhodes, A. Y., and Ormsby, H. L. Tissue culture techniques in the study of herpetic infections of the eye, Am. J. Ophth., 40 (Part 2): 189, 1957.

8. Gallardo, E. Primary herpes simplex keratitis; clinical and experimental study, Arch. Ophth., 30:217, 1943.

9. Hanna, L., Jawetz, E., and Coleman, V. R. The significance of isolating herpes simplex virus from the eye, Am. J. Ophth., 43 (Part 2): 126, 1957.

10. Hogan, M. J. Corneal transplantation in the treatment of herpetic disease of the cornea, Am. J. Ophth., 43 (Part 2):147, 1957.

11. Howard, G. M., and Kaufman, H. E. Herpes simplex keratitis: Special reviews, Arch. Ophth., 67:373, 1962.

12. Kaufman, H. E., Nesburn, A. B., and Maloney, E. D. IDU therapy of herpes simplex, Arch. Ophth., 67:583, 1962.

13. Kimura, S. J., and Okumoto, M. A. The effect of corticosteroids on experimental herpes simplex keratoconjunctivitis in the rabbit, Am. J. Ophth., 43 (Part 2):131, 1957.

14. Lennette, E. H., and van Allen, A. Laboratory diagnosis of herpetic infections of the eye, Am. J. Ophth., 43 (Part 2):118, 1957.

15. Ormsby, H. L. Superficial forms of herpetic keratitis, Am. J. Ophth., 43 (Part 2): 107, 1957.

16. Rake, G. W. The etiologic role of the virus of herpes simplex in ophthalmic disease, Am. J. Ophth., 43 (Part 2):113, 1957.

17. Scott, T. F. M., Coriell, L. L., Blank, H., and Gray, A. The growth curve of the virus of herpes simplex on the chorioallantoic membrane of the embryonated hen's egg, J. Immunol., 71:134, 1953.

18. Thomas, C. I. The Cornea, Springfield, Ill., Charles C Thomas, Publisher, 1955.

19. Thygeson, P., Hogan, M. J., and Kimura, S. J. Cortisone and hydrocortisone in ocular infections, Tr. Am. Acad. Ophth., 57:64, 1953.

20. ——— Kimura, S. J., and Hogan, M. J. Observations on herpetic keratitis and keratoconjunctivitis, Arch. Ophth., 56:375, 1956.

21. ——— and Kimura, S. J. Deep forms of herpetic keratitis, Am. J. Ophth., 43 (Part 2):109, 1957.

VARICELLA-HERPES ZOSTER GROUP
(Shingles, Herpes Zoster, Zona)

Herpes zoster and herpes simplex have been proven, antigenically and clinically, to be different viruses. Therefore, since the term herpes zoster may be confusing, it seems better to use only the term zoster.

Zoster is believed by many to be related to the varicella virus, but this concept is still controversial. Cultural and serologic investigation led Weller to the conclusion that the zoster and varicella viruses are identical.[8] It has been shown that inoculation of zoster vesicle fluid into infants causes varicella-like diseases, but not in children convalescing from varicella. However, adults frequently initiate epidemics of varicella.[1] The relationship between these two viruses is probably analogous to that of herpes simplex with its primary or recurrent forms. Varicella is a primary manifestation in children; then the virus becomes latent, localized within nerve cells. Various stimulating factors, such as breast cancer, leukemia, intramuscular injections, trauma, or others, can cause the latent viruses to be manifested as zoster. In patients with zoster it is also advisable to check for leukemia or breast cancer.

Clinical Features. Zoster is characterized by skin or mucous membrane vesicular lesions distributed along one or more groups of sensory nerves; simultaneously, the dorsal roots of the trunk or dorsal ganglia are involved. Zoster is most frequently manifested on the neck, shoulders, and arms, the process usually being unilateral. The incubation period is not fully established. Severe pain is typical at the onset of the condition; then vesicles appear. They become ulcerated and covered by crusts. Scarring may ensue. Early in the disease the lymph nodes of the involved area are enlarged. Persistent neuralgia in older subjects is usual in convalescence.

Clinical features of varicella are subjects for the pediatrician and therefore will not be discussed here. Ocular involvements are rare, but vesicles are nearly always present on the lid as part of the general skin eruption. Temporary blindness may be associated with an encephalitis, which is an occasional complication of varicella. It must be emphasized that steroid therapy should be avoided. Fatal results have been reported, especially when the varicella was complicated by pneumonia.[4]

Findings in the Eye. Zoster ophthalmicus is usually an acute unilateral and severe process characterized by vesicular eruptions along the ophthalmic branches of the trigeminus nerve (Plate XXVI, 1). Frequently the gasserian ganglion is inflamed; this is the symptomatic zoster. The vesicles occur at the inner half of the lid if the supratrochlear branch is involved. If the nasociliar branch is attacked, keratitis may result. This is manifested mainly as subepithelial, discrete infiltrates, or in the form of a disc in the epithelium consisting of punctate dots. Simultaneously, vesicles in rows or groups are occasionally seen (Plate XXVI, 3). They rupture rapidly, forming superficial ulcers. Neuroparalytic keratitis may develop in more severe cases. These ulcers may be easily complicated by secondary bacterial infection, resulting in hypopyon keratitis. Interstitial disciform keratitis, although rare, appears mainly as a severe process, accompanied by Descemet's folds (Plate XXVI, 2). It develops within one or more weeks after the onset of zoster and is probably of allergenic origin. Disciform keratitis is frequently complicated by iridocyclitis and glaucoma. In any of these keratitides, scarring and a marked decrease of sensitivity are typical.

The diagnosis of ocular zoster is determined by the presence of typical skin manifestations.

Involvement of the eye in chickenpox is rare. A mild conjunctivitis or vesicular keratitis may occur. These are usually associated with lid eruptions and disappear rapidly (Plate XXVI, 5). When varicella-zoster virus diseases are complicated by encephalitis, ocular motor paralyses are frequent. The optic nerve is rarely affected.

Laboratory Studies. The virus has not been found to produce disease in any species other than man. It was first transmitted to volunteers (children) by Steiner.[7] Weller first grew viruses of varicella and zoster in the cell culture of human embryonic tissue. He found that both viruses produced had the same type of cytopathogenic effect. Goodpasture and Anderson [2] accomplished growth of the zoster virus in skin grafted on the chorioallantois of chick embryos. Fluorescent antibody technic gave evidence of the mutual antibody relationship of the varicella and zoster viruses.

Intranuclear Lipschütz inclusion bodies, similar to those of herpes simplex are found. Their relationship to virus multiplication is not sufficiently clear, as similar inclusion bodies have appeared in some nonviral conditions. The development of inclusion bodies is the same as in herpes simplex (see page 125). Ballooning cell degeneration, giant multinucleated cells, and many polymorphonuclear cells are also found (Plate XXVI, 4).

Immunity. Both varicella and zoster usually produce a lasting immunity. Nevertheless the varicella virus may remain localized and latent, but under certain conditions it can be reactivated. The mechanism of the phenomenon is not clear.

Treatment. Treatment is symptomatic. The eruptions of zoster and varicella require care in the prevention of secondary bacterial infection. If such infection has already developed, sulfonamides and the proper antibiotics are used. Personal hygiene, especially of the skin, is an important measure. Sedative ointments are indicated in severe pain. Section of the sensory root may be required if chronic neuralgia develops.

REFERENCES

1. Amies, C. R.   The elementary bodies of zoster and their serological relationship to those of varicella, Brit. J. Exper. Path., 15:314, 1934.
2. Goodpasture, E. W., and Anderson, K.   Infection of human skin, grafted on the chorioallantois of chick embryos, with the virus of herpes zoster, Am. J. Path., 20:447, 1944.
3. Griffin, W. P., and Searle, C. W. A.   Ocular manifestations of varicella, Lancet, 2:168, 1953.
4. Haggerty, R. J., and Eley, R. C.   Varicella and cortisone (Letter to Editor), Pediatrics, 18:160, 1956.
5. Lipschütz, B.   Untersuchungen über die Ätiologie der Krankheiten der Herpesgruppe (Herpes zoster, Herpes genitalis, Herpes febrilis), Arch. Dermat. u. Syph., 136:428, 1921.
6. Rivers, T. M.   Nuclear inclusions in the testicles of monkeys injected with the tissue of human varicella lesions, J. Exper. Med., 43:275, 1926.
7. Steiner, G.   Zur inokulation varicellen, Wien. Med. Wchnschr., 25:306, 1875.
8. Weller, T. H.   Serial propagation in vitro of agents producing inclusion bodies derived from varicella and herpes zoster, Proc. Soc. Exper. Biol. & Med., 83:340, 1953.
9. ───── and Coons, A. H.   Fluorescent antibody studies with agents of varicella and herpes zoster propagated in vitro, Proc. Soc. Exper. Biol. & Med., 86:789, 1954.

ADENOVIRUS GROUP

Adenoviruses are the most recently described group of medically important viruses, having been isolated by tissue culture technics. The first isolation was reported by Rowe and his co-workers in 1953.[11] The agents, found in fragments of surgically removed human adenoids, were initially called adenoid degeneration viruses. Almost simultaneously, Hilleman and Werner,[2] also by tissue culture technic, isolated a virus from Army recruits having acute respiratory disease (ARD). In the same year Huebner studied a clinical entity for which he suggested the name adeno-pharyngeal-conjunctivitis (APC).[3] The name adenovirus proposed by Enders et al.[1] has been generally accepted since 1956.

Adenovirus infection is world-wide, causing mainly respiratory tract and eye diseases—acute respiratory diseases (ARD) and pharyngoconjunctival fever (PCF). ARD and PCF often occur in epidemic form and have some clinical symptoms in common. These include fever and lymphadenopathy.

Findings in the Eye. Following isolation of adenoviruses, intensive studies of the eye involvements were made, particularly in the United States (Jawetz, Thygeson, Kimura, Hogan et al.), and Japan (Mitsui, Tanka, Kumano et al.).*

Various adenoviral eye infections are now distinguished. The most common adenoviral infection of children is PCF. This is characterized by the triad: pharyngitis, conjunctivitis, and fever. The incubation period is from two to ten days. Mild pharyngitis is accompanied by adenopathy, usually submaxillary. It is often associated with high fever, even to 104°F. The child may have coryza, gastrointestinal disturbances, or meningismus.

The conjunctivitis is follicular, often unilateral, and usually involves the lower fornix. It lasts about three weeks. The other eye may become involved, usually not so severely, two to five days after onset of the condition. A superficial transitory corneal opacity may be present. Serologic Type 3 is the principal cause of PCF.

Epidemics of PCF usually occur during the summer, infecting children 4 to 9 years old. Swimming pools may be a source of infection.

The PCF triad in epidemic form is virtually pathognomonic for adenoviral infection, as the clinical picture is more constant and characteristic in epidemics. More difficult to diagnose are the sporadic cases of PCF. Without laboratory confirmation the diagnosis is only tentative. Sporadic cases of PCF have been studied by Kimura et al.[6] These have mainly involved adults, and in a less severe form than in children. Type 3 adenovirus was isolated from PCF in about half of the cases studied; Types 2 and 6 were occasionally found.

Apart from the triad, adenovirus can cause follicular conjunctivitis without systemic symptoms or sore throat. The preauricular nodes (not maxillary as in PCF) are enlarged and tender. The infection occurs in epidemic form, the source usually being swimming pools. We have seen several other-

* Adenoviruses are thoroughly discussed in the Proceedings of a Symposium on Viral Keratoconjunctivitis, *Am. J. Ophth.*, Vol. 43, No. 4, Part 2, April, 1957.

wise asymptomatic patients with follicular conjunctivitis in which adenovirus Type 3 was isolated. They usually occurred in the winter, either sporadically or in small epidemics. Without isolation of the virus, these cases
represent a diagnostic problem easily confused with herpetic follicular conjunctivitis. Important points of differentiation are skin eruptions or acute
blepharitis in herpetic infections.

Epidemic keratoconjunctivitis (EKC), another classical triad, has recently been shown to be caused by an adenovirus. The first strain of adenovirus Type 8 was isolated from epidemic keratoconjunctivitis by Jawetz
et al.; these investigators were also first to isolate a strain of adenovirus from
follicular conjunctivitis. A number of epidemics had already established
EKC as a clinical entity. Since these epidemics occurred among shipyard
employees, the triad was called the shipyard disease. Later observations
showed that these endemics or epidemics can affect many other persons.
Instrument transmission, especially by tonometer, must be avoided.

Classically, a follicular conjunctivitis in the lower fornix initiates the
process. Edema of the semilunar fold and caruncula, chemosis, petechiae,
and ecchymosis may develop. Systemic involvement is usually lacking.

The keratitis, which follows 7 to 10 days after onset of the conjunctivitis,
is characterized by small, round, discrete, grayish subepithelial infiltrates.
The keratitis typically localizes in the pupillary area and may last two to
eight weeks or even longer. As a rule it clears without sequelae.

The triad is considered pathognomonic for diagnosis. However, Japa-
nese observers [8, 12] have described a form of EKC in infants which has atypical manifestations. These include a membranous type of conjunctivitis accompanied by systemic symptoms. Most interesting and surprising is the fact
that the cornea was not involved; Type 8 was, however, isolated. These observers believed the epidemic resulted from swimming pool transmission.

The term EKC has been confused further because diagnosis is often
based only on the typical subepithelial, punctate, central keratitis. Therefore,
in such cases the term subepithelial adenoviral keratitis would be more appropriate. Then this picture could be regarded as pathognomonic in analogy with herpetic dendritic keratitis.

Laboratory Studies. Most attempts to produce adenoviral infections in
laboratory animals have failed. Man appears to be the only host for most
adenoviruses. Transmission to volunteers has often been positive,[14] especially in the case of conjunctivitis. Mitsui produced keratitis in volunteers
by inoculation of Type 8 isolated from EKC.[7]

Cultivation of adenoviruses has been successful in HeLa cells, monkey
kidney tissue, and rabbit trachea epithelial cells. Inclusion bodies have been
found in positive tissue culture. They are eosinophilic, and are initially
Feulgen-negative, later becoming basophilic Feulgen-positive. The electron
microscope shows viral particles in crystalline arrangement.

Adenoviruses have been studied, and as a result at least 23 serologic types are known; of these, 18 are human parasites sharing many serologic and biologic properties. Hence similar diseases and epidemics are produced by different antigenic types. It is also true that in an epidemic more than one serologic type may be present.

Most of the adenovirus isolations have been from adenoids and tonsils which often harbor several serologic types. Their causative role in adenoid hypertrophy has not been proven. Possibly this adenoid tissue serves as a reservoir for latent adenoviruses.

Although there is no constant relationship between the type of virus and the induced disease, one usually finds a predominant type in the epidemic, endemic, or sporadic cases. Types 3 and 7 are epidemic strains in persons of all ages. Types 1 and 2 are endemic strains which are highly contagious.[10] They infect the majority of children before the age of 2 or 3 years and persist in the adenoids and tonsils. Types 3, 4, 5, 6, and 7 more commonly infect adults. Type 4 is found in acute respiratory diseases of adults, while Types 1 and 2 are found in children. In ocular disease, Type 3 is a common finding in follicular conjunctivitis and Type 8 in EKC (Jawetz). The variation of serologic types is particularly evident in sporadic cases. In epidemics, the clinical picture and relation to serologic types are usually more constant. Further serologic study is needed for clarification. According to recent data, it would appear that all important serologic types fall into only two major subgroups. The duration of immunity has not been determined.

To determine the specific virus type which caused the infection, neutralization titration must be done with the common types of adenoviruses known to cause infection (Rivers and Horsfall).[9]

Treatment. Antibiotics, convalescent serum, and virus vaccination have no value in treating adenovirus infection. The treatment is symptomatic. Hot compresses and mydriatics, when indicated, give some relief. The principal care must be to increase the patient's general resistance by such factors as sufficient vitamin intake, proper diet, and rest. Any stresses and disturbances of the physical and physiologic balance—including indiscriminate use of new medicines—should be avoided. Variation of seasons, range of age, irritation of mucous membranes, or trauma may be significant contributory factors. Extreme care must be used in cleaning instruments, especially the tonometer.[13]

Vaccination or injection of gamma globulin may be useful in preventing epidemics. Special epidemiologic circumstances should be decided by an epidemiologist.

REFERENCES

1. Enders, J. F., Bell, J. A., Dingle, J. H., Francis, T., Jr., Hilleman, M. R., Huebner, R. J., and Payne, A. M. "Adenoviruses": Group name proposed for new respiratory-tract viruses, Science, 124:119, 1956.

2. Hilleman, M. R., and Werner, J. H.   Recovery of new agent from patients with acute respiratory illness, Proc. Soc. Exper. Biol. & Med., 85:183, 1954.
3. Huebner, R. J., Rowe, W. P., Ward, T. G., Parrott, R. H., and Bell, J. A.   Adenoidal-pharyngeal-conjunctival agents. A newly recognized group of common viruses of the respiratory system, New England J. Med., 251:1077, 1954.
4. Jawetz, E., Kimura, S., Nicholas, A. N., Thygeson, P., and Hanna, L.   New type of APC virus from epidemic keratoconjunctivitis, Science, 122:1190, 1955.
5. ——— Hanna, L., Kimura, S. J., and Thygeson, P.   A new type of APC virus from follicular conjunctivitis, Am. J. Ophth., 41:231, 1956.
6. Kimura, S. J., Hanna, M. A., Nicholas, B. A., Thygeson, P., and Jawetz, E.   Sporadic cases of pharyngoconjunctival fever in northern California, 1955-1956, Am. J. Ophth., 43(Part 2):14, 1957.
7. Mitsui, Y., Hanabusa, J., Minoda, R., and Ogata, S.   Effect of inoculating adenovirus (APC virus) type 8 into human volunteers, Am. J. Ophth., 43(Part 2):84, 1957.
8. ——— and Jawetz, E.   Isolation of adenovirus type 8 (APC type 8) from a case of epidemic keratoconjunctivitis in Japan, Am. J. Ophth., 43(Part 2):91, 1957.
9. Rivers, T. M., and Horsfall, F. L.   Viral and Rickettsial Infections of Man, 3rd ed., Philadelphia, J. B. Lippincott Co., 1959.
10. Rose, H. M., editor.   Viral Infections of Infancy and Childhood, New York, Paul B. Hoeber, Inc., 1960.
11. Rowe, W. P., Huebner, R. J., Gilmore, L. K., Parrott, R. H., and Ward, T. G.   Isolation of a cytopathogenic agent from human adenoids undergoing spontaneous degenerations in tissue culture, Proc. Soc. Exper. Biol. & Med., 84:570, 1953.
12. Tanaka, C.   Epidemic keratoconjunctivitis in Japan and the Orient.   Paper given at Keratoconjunctivitis Symposium, San Francisco, Sept. 7-8, 1956.
13. Thygeson, P.   Office and dispensary transmissions of epidemic keratoconjunctivitis, Am. J. Ophth., 43(Part 2):98, 1957.
14. Ward, T. G., Huebner, R. J., Rowe, W. P., Ryan, R. W., and Bell, J. A.   Production of pharyngoconjunctival fever in human volunteers inoculated with APC viruses, Science, 122:1086, 1955.

MEASLES

Measles, an infectious exanthematous disease usually of childhood, occurs in epidemic form. In debilitated patients and those of low resistance, or when secondary infection occurs (most often *H. influenzae,* staphylococci, or streptococci), the disease can be fatal. The commonest bacterial complications are otitis media with perforation of the drum, or bronchopneumonia. Acute catarrhal conjunctivitis is commonly present. Measles encephalomyelitis is uncommon; it has a high mortality and may cause permanent neurologic damage. Also, measles infection may possibly lower the body's resistance to other infections such as tuberculosis.

One attack of measles usually confers lifelong immunity; nevertheless recurrent cases, especially in adults, have been reported.

Clinical Findings.   The incubation period for measles is about 14 days. The prodromal period, the most contagious, is characterized by fever and catarrhal symptoms: conjunctivitis, cough, running nose, and sneezing. Koplik's spots are important for early diagnosis of measles and differentiate measles from rubella.[2] They are bluish white, surrounded by scarlet red areolas, and typically localized around the papillae of the parotid duct. However, other mucous membranes including the conjunctiva may be involved. These spots represent necrosis of epithelium. The prodromal period lasts from one to five days and is followed by the typical eruption.

Findings in the Eye. Usually mild, acute catarrhal, nonpurulent conjunctivitis commonly develops. It is characterized by a severe photophobia; occasionally marked edema of the conjunctiva is present. The conjunctivitis is thought to be caused by the virus. The process usually subsides when desquamation of the skin begins, but in cases complicated by bacterial infection, severe purulent conjunctivitis may be observed throughout the entire illness. In debilitated children, a severe true membranous conjunctivitis may occur. Koplik's spots have been found on the conjunctiva and on the lacrimal caruncula (cited from Duke-Elder). Lid margins may become red and swollen during the conjunctivitis or in the period of eruption. Infectious suppurative inflammation of the meibomian glands sometimes complicates this blepharitis. Gangrene of the lids rarely occurs.

Keratitis is not a usual complication, and when it occurs it is mainly a punctate superficial type. This may ulcerate and vascularize. In cases with bacterial contamination the keratitis becomes purulent, sometimes followed by panophthalmitis and phthisis bulbi. Metastatic uveitis may occasionally occur.

Laboratory Studies. The measles virus host range is limited. It has been transmitted to susceptible species of monkeys.[1] Cultivation of the virus is difficult, but tissue cultivation has recently been achieved in monkey and dog kidney tissue. Growth has also been successful on chick embryo chorio-allantoic membrane (Rake and Shaffer).[4]

Enders and Peebles in 1960 reported positive growth in tissue culture of human kidney cells.

Cytology. Multinucleated giant cells in the sputum and nasal mucosa during the prodromal period are diagnostically important. In experiments, the giant cells have been found to contain eosinophilic intranuclear inclusion bodies and cytoplasmic eosinophilic masses. Similar inclusion bodies have been described in human specimens (Torres in Blank and Rake).[2] In measles infection, one finds a monocytic cellular response; the monocytes contain cytoplasmic granules which may be hyalin.

Treatment. This is usually symptomatic; warm saline to keep the eye clean is recommended. To relieve the photophobia in cases of conjunctivitis, it is better to keep the patient out of direct light. Antibiotics are necessary in cases of secondary bacterial infection. Gamma globulin together with live vaccine may be effective, particularly in preventing encephalitis. The Enders measles vaccine may eventually eliminate this disease, thus solving the problem of its severe complications.

REFERENCES

1. Anderson, J. F., and Goldberger, J.   Experimental measles in the monkey; a sup-
    plemental note, Pub. Health Rep., 26:887, 1911.
2. Blank, H., and Rake, G.   Viral and Rickettsial Diseases of the Skin, Eye and
    Mucous Membranes of Man, Boston, Little, Brown & Co., 1955.
3. Doggart, J. H.   Affections of the eye with relation to skin diseases, Brit. M. J.,
    2:792, 1937.
4. Rake, G., and Shaffer, M. F.   Propagation of the agent of measles in the fertile hen's
    egg, Nature, 144:672, 1939.

MUMPS
(Epidemic Parotitis)

Mumps is a contagious viral disease. Its viral origin was proven in 1934 by Johnson and Goodpasture. Epidemics of mumps are frequent, especially in military establishments. While the commonest manifestation is parotitis, other organs such as the pancreas, ovaries, or testicles may also be primarily affected. Hence, rather than "complications," the term manifestations is more accurate. Mumps is now regarded as a viremia rather than a localized infection of the salivary glands.

Many cases of ocular involvement have been reported.

Clinical Features.   The salivary manifestations usually occur in children aged 5 to 13 years. The incubation period is 18 to 21 days, after which one or both parotids swell; there are accompanying fever and headache. Swelling of the submaxillary glands is often present. The portal of entry is usually the respiratory tract, but the conjunctival epithelium may be the primary site for multiplication of the virus. The virus may spread via the blood stream into certain parts of the body, including the eye; then symptoms appear. The disease may be complicated by generalized viremia and often by meningoencephalitis.

Mumps, while often symptomatic, may be symptomless.

Findings in the Eye.   The most recent and complete review of ocular manifestations of the mumps virus is by Riffenburgh.[5] Dacryoadenitis and optic neuritis most commonly occur. In epidemic mumps, dacryoadenitis may precede the parotitis.[2, 3] The onset of dacryoadenitis is sudden, painful, and usually bilateral. Its duration is several weeks, and healing is without sequelae.

Optic neuritis or papillitis is usually benign; only rarely does optic atrophy occur.[7] Corneal infection is also frequent, particularly during the febrile period (Danielson and Long).[1] The most common corneal picture presents as an unusual unilateral interstitial keratitis (Nectoux).[4] This keratitis is characterized by a dense opacity which may rapidly progress to involve the entire cornea. Occasionally only one quadrant is affected. Numerous folds in Descemet's membrane are evident. The process disappears spontaneously, usually within two weeks, leaving no trace. This typical picture is regarded as pathognomonic for mumps. It may be associated with anterior uveitis. Occasionally a punctate ulcerative or nodular keratitis, resembling nummular keratitis, is seen. The other ocular manifestations, not infrequent, are conjunctivitis (usually without secretion), benign episcleritis, and scleritis.

Rare ocular manifestations are central retinal vein occlusion and congenital abnormalities following mumps infection of the mother during the early months of pregnancy.[6]

Treatment. The treatment is symptomatic. Concentrated normal gamma globulin has proved to be of no value. Several steroid hormones have been used. However, their value is not established.

REFERENCES

1. Danielson, R. W., and Long, J. C. Keratitis due to mumps, Am. J. Ophth., 24:655, 1941.
2. Galpine, J. F., and Walkowski, J. A case of mumps with involvement of the lacrimal glands, Brit. M. J., 1:1069, 1952.
3. Jones, B. R. Clinical features and aetiology of dacryoadenitis, Tr. Ophth. Soc. U. Kingdom, 75:435, 1955.
4. Nectoux, R. Keratite ourlienne, Ann. ocul., 179:597, 1946.
5. Riffenburgh, R. D. Ocular manifestations of mumps. Special reviews, Arch. Ophth., 66:739, 1961.
6. Siegel, M., and Greenberg, M. Virus diseases in pregnancy and their effects on the fetus, Am. J. Obst. & Gynec., 77:620, 1959.
7. Swab, C. M. Encephalitic optic neuritis and atrophy due to mumps, Arch. Ophth., 19:926, 1938.

MOLLUSCUM CONTAGIOSUM

Molluscum contagiosum was recognized as a clinical entity as early as 1817 (van Rooyen and Rhodes).[18] It is common in Edinburgh, Scotland, but sporadic or epidemic occurrence is known in many parts of the world. The infection is spread by direct or indirect contact (i.e., barbers, common towels, scratching). Swimming pools are one source of infection. Pigeons, dogs, and other domestic animals may develop molluscum and contaminate man.

Molluscum contagiosum is a local disease of mild infectivity. Its most interesting feature is the architecture of the molluscum body, once considered a protozoan parasite. However, these are now recognized as viral bodies; study with the electron microscope has added knowledge of their detailed structure.

Clinical Features. Molluscum contagiosum is mainly a childhood disease, characterized by benign epithelial nodules on any part of the skin, especially the facial. Mucous membranes of the genitalia are often involved. Lesions are uninflamed, round, waxy, and white. The summit is usually umbilicated, having a tiny black spot. Cheesy masses consisting of degenerated epithelial cells can readily be expressed. The typical lesions are easily diagnosed—however, sometimes they appear in atypical forms: sebaceous cyst, verruca, or milium (Curtin and Theodore).[5]

Findings in the Eye. Ocular manifestation of molluscum contagiosum is primarily on the lid skin. The lesions vary in size from very small to giganteum (Meer Maastricht) [12] and number from one to a dozen, sometimes grouped in semiconfluented masses (Plate XXIX, 1). Suppuration due to secondary infection may occur. The lesions occasionally disappear spontaneously.

Various ocular manifestations due to extension of the skin molluscum have been described. Reviews of the literature are given by Duke-Elder,[6] Lee,[9] and others.[10, 11, 16] If the lesion is situated at the lid margin, conjunctivitis or keratitis or both may develop. The conjunctivitis is usually a chronic, recurrent, follicular type, with considerable papillary hypertrophy and thickening of the conjunctiva. The picture resembles trachoma.

Several types of keratitis, independent or associated with the conjunctivitis, may develop: epithelial, punctate, marginal, or pannus. The pannus (Plate XXIX, 2) involves the upper part of the cornea and thus resembles trachomatous pannus. The presence of molluscum contagiosum at the margin and the absence of trachomatous inclusion bodies are diagnostic aids. The complication disappears after removal of the lid lesion; toxic or mechanical origin may therefore be considered. Nevertheless, direct viral invasion may occur, causing conjunctival or corneal phlyctenule-like nodules.

Laboratory Studies. Numerous attempts to cultivate the virus have failed. Animal inoculation experiments have also been negative.[15] Man is the only known host.

The virus is plentiful in individual skin lesions and can readily be demonstrated by the electron microscope (Banfield et al.).[2] This is one of the largest viruses, and its shape is ovoid.

The cytoplasmic, eosinophilic inclusion bodies, described by Henderson [8] and Paterson,[14] were later shown to be composed of elementary bodies. Several stages of their development have been described. In the mature stage, the eosinophilic globular masses, separated by septa, represent aggregations of elementary bodies. The nucleus, pushed to the wall, becomes almost invisible (Plate XXIX, 3).

There is no evidence of immunity.

No specific treatment exists. Surgery is usually the best approach; however, electrocoagulation may be preferred for lid margin lesions.

WARTS
(Verruca, Skin Papilloma)

Warts are horny growths on the skin and, rarely, mucous membranes. They may occur as a primary invasion of the lids, particularly the lid margins. However, transmission from other body areas is a more common occurrence. Animals may be affected and can be a source of infection for man.

Thorough studies and references are given by Blank and Rake.[3] Various clinical types, distinguished by structure, localization, age of patient, and other clinical features, are: common warts (verruca vulgaris), flat warts (verruca plantaris), filiform warts (verruca filiformis), moist warts (venereal warts), and flat, greasy warts seen in the elderly (verruca senilis).

All warts are believed to be caused by a single virus. Verruca vulgaris, the most frequent type, is commonly seen in children. Girls are more subject to verruca plantaris than are boys or adults. Moist warts may be found on the conjunctiva, although they usually involve the genitalia. This type undergoes malignant changes more frequently than the others. Filiform warts are the commonest wart of the lid skin and lid margins.

Like molluscum contagiosum, the wart virus is slow-growing and of mild infectivity. The incubation period is from 1 to 20 months. The infection spreads by direct or indirect contact (i.e., barbers, common towels, shaking hands, communal washing facilities, bathing pools, or venereal contact). Warts are less common in the United States than in Europe. However, incidence is increasing in crowded military installations and in areas having poor hygiene.

Findings in the Eye. Filiform warts may involve the lid skin and are frequently associated with lesions of the bearded area, disseminated by shaving (Plate XXIX, 5). Rarely, cornu cutaneum, a horn-shaped excrescence, may appear. An unusually long cornu cutaneum (about 3 cm) at the inner lid canthus was observed by the author (Plate XXIX, 4).

Filiform and common warts, the most frequent lid margin warts, are slowly progressive. They may be single or coalescent and develop between the lashes, usually of the upper lids.

Conjunctivitis, keratitis, or even corneal ulceration may occasionally complicate lid margin warts. In contrast to molluscum contagiosum, the conjunctivitis is a subacute catarrhal type and is not follicular. Duke-Elder and Thygeson have emphasized that the keratitis is strictly epithelial and often occurs without conjunctivitis. Considerable pain and photophobia are characteristic, and recurrence is frequent. A vascular type of keratitis somewhat like rosacea keratitis may occur. The exact mechanism of these complications is unknown. However, in analogy with molluscum contagiosum, a toxic, allergic, or mechanical origin may be assumed.

Additionally, it seems appropriate to mention the role of bacteria; the rough surface of the wart may become a locus for bacterial growth. Conjunctivitis or superficial keratitis can ensue from the infection itself or from bacterial sensitization.

Laboratory Studies. Warts are infective, as proved long ago by inoculation of volunteers (Variot, 1894)[19] and by self-inoculation (Ciuffo, 1907).[4] This was more fully confirmed and expanded by Wile and Kingery (1919)[20] and Goodman and Greenwood (1934).[7] Practically all of the experimental work has been done with human volunteers. Numerous attempts to transmit warts to animals have failed or have lacked confirmation.

Cytologic study in the past was confusing. The structures seen in the granular layer, such as keratohyalin granules, were once regarded as inclusion bodies. Later, the specific structures were recognized as the real inclusion bodies. Their positive Feulgen reaction confirms that they are newly formed DNA. The cells showing ballooning degeneration of the cytoplasm are called "bird's-eye cells." Studies with the electron microscope by Strauss et al.[17] and Melnick et al.[13] added significant knowledge concerning structure of the inclusion bodies, demonstrating a virus aggregation having the appearance of crystals.

Treatment.   There is no specific or uniform treatment; every case must be individualized.

Surgical removal is often successful. However, the lesion may recur on the scar. Chemical destruction is usually effective and simple. Trichloracetic acid, silver nitrate pencil, nitric acid, and salicylic acid have been successfully used.

Psychotherapy or suggestion therapy is widely accepted. Wart charmers use various mystical procedures (cited from Blank and Rake). An extensive review of psychotherapy was made by Allington in 1952.[1] Many agree that none of the chemical and physical methods are better than suggestion.

Spontaneous disappearance of warts has been observed.

REFERENCES

1. Allington, H. V.   Review of the psychotherapy of warts, Arch. Dermat., 66:316, 1952.
2. Banfield, W. G., Bunting, H., Strauss, M. J., and Melnick, J. L.   Electronmicrographs of thin sections of molluscum contagiosum, Proc. Soc. Exper. Biol. & Med., 77:843, 1951.
3. Blank, H., and Rake, G.   Viral and Rickettsial Diseases of the Skin, Eye and Mucous Membranes of Man, Boston, Little, Brown & Co., 1955.
4. Ciuffo, G.   Innesto positivo con filtrato di verruca volgare, Gior. ital. d. mal. ven., 48:12, 1907.
5. Curtin, B. J., and Theodore, F. H.   Ocular molluscum contagiosum, Am. J. Ophth., 39:302, 1955.
6. Duke-Elder, W. S.   Text-book of Ophthalmology, St. Louis, Mo., C. V. Mosby Co., 1946, vol. 2, pp. 1738-1739.
7. Goodman, J., Jr., and Greenwood, A. M.   Verrucae, a review, Arch. Dermat., 30:659, 1934.
8. Henderson, W.   Edinburgh M. & S. J., 56:213, 1841.
9. Lee, O. S., Jr.   Keratitis occurring with molluscum contagiosum, Arch. Ophth., 31:64, 1944.
10. Magnus, J. A.   Unilateral follicular conjunctivitis due to molluscum contagiosum, Brit. J. Ophth., 28:245, 1944.
11. Mathur, S. P.   Ocular complications in molluscum contagiosum, Brit. J. Ophth., 44:572, 1960.

12. Meer Maastricht, B.C.J.v.d., and Gomperts, C. E.   Molluscum contagiosum giganteum, Am. J. Ophth., 33:965, 1950.

13. Melnick, J. L., Bunting, H., Banfield, W. G., Strauss, M. J., and Gaylord, W. H. Electron microscopy of viruses of human papilloma molluscum contagiosum and vaccinia, including observations on the formation of virus within the cell, Ann. New York Acad. Sc., 54:1214, 1952.

14. Paterson, R.   Edinburgh M. & S. J., 56:279, 1841.

15. Rake, G., and Blank, H.   The relationship of host and virus in molluscum contagiosum, J. Invest. Dermat., 15:81, 1950.

16. Rocha, H.   Molluscum contagiosum (abstract), Am. J. Ophth, 27:929, 1944.

17. Strauss, M. J., Bunting, H., and Melnick, J. L.   Virus-like particles and inclusion bodies in skin papillomas, J. Invest. Dermat., 15:433, 1950.

18. van Rooyen, C. E., and Rhodes, A. J.   Virus Diseases of Man, 2nd ed., New York, Thomas Nelson Sons, 1948.

19. Variot, G.   Un cas d'inoculation expérimentale des verrues de l'enfant à l'homme, J. clin. et thérap. inf. (Paris), 2:529, 1894.

20. Wile, U. J., and Kingery, L. B.   The etiology of common warts, J.A.M.A., 73:970, 1919.

4

Fungi

SOME GENERAL ASPECTS

Fungi are important both as vectors of disease and as agents for industrial fermentation. Vegetable organisms of low order, they are structurally more complicated than bacteria, being larger, vacuolized, and usually having a sexual mechanism. Lacking chlorophyll, they are not photosynthetic. The soil is their most common environment, and they are a leading cause of plant disease.

Many of the fungi which act as laboratory contaminants were considered nonpathogenic. Recent studies reveal that some of these so-called nonpathogenic fungi may cause severe, even fatal, diseases in man. Of over 1,000 species of fungi, 50 or more may infect man and animals. The type of mycosis and its distribution vary geographically.

Mycotic diseases, including those of the eye, appear to be on the rise since the advent of antibiotics and steroids, as well as increased therapeutic use of nitrogen mustard.

As descriptions of fungi are complex and specialized, the ophthalmologist need not be acquainted with a detailed study. Only the practical general aspects will be discussed herein. Some details will be given in the description of specific disease entities of ocular importance.

Morphology.   Fungi are usually multicellular, filamentous structures, although yeasts and some branched fungi are unicellular. A hypha is an individual filament; a mass of hyphae constitute the mycelium, which is better demonstrated in the culture. Mycelia can also be shown in superficial mycoses of the skin or mucous membranes.

Fungi are gram-positive; some are acid-fast and can be mistaken for tubercle bacilli. Staining is usually uneven, creating a granular appearance. Most fungi possess cell walls and vacuoles; special staining demonstrates these. The filaments of some fungi fragment easily into bacillary and coccoid elements.

Microscopic examination of original clinical material is important and may lead to diagnosis of mycosis more readily than does the culture.

Culture. Fungi grow readily on most routine laboratory media aerobically and at room temperature. On media, fungus growth is slow, usually taking more than one week. The culture must be prevented from drying. Sabouraud's medium is the most satisfactory for fungi. However, special media and methods are needed to identify certain species. The cultures show a great variation of appearance, even on the same medium. Therefore, identification is not easy. The filamentous colonies are usually powdery, cottony, prickly, or with a leathery consistency. The growth has a marked tendency to spread over the surface of the medium.

Yeast colonies are soft, bacterialike, consisting only of budding cells (e.g., *Cryptococcus*). Yeastlike colonies are also soft, but besides the budding cells on the surface of the medium, there are hyphae which penetrate it (e.g., in *Candida* species).

Examination of the Fungi. Fungi are identified on the basis of the type of spores and their arrangement. Several special methods are used to prepare specimens for spore examination. For some species, the tube or plate is placed on the stage and examined, using the low-power objective. This must be done carefully without disturbing the growth. Then the hyphae and spores can be seen. There are two types of hyphae: vegetative, to secure food, and fertile, to produce spores. Some filamentous fungi are examined in a drop of mounting medium on the slide. The filaments must be carefully teased with needles, then covered by a coverglass. Lactophenol cotton blue, glycerin, or eosin can be used as a mounting medium. The yeastlike colonies are best examined by emulsifying a bit of the colony in a drop of water and preparing the usual wet slide. Skin, hair, and nails should be examined on a slide with a drop of 10 per cent potassium hydroxide. It is best to heat the slide before examination, to clarify the specimen. Exudates or other direct specimens are usually examined as fresh preparations or may be stained by various methods.

Extreme caution should be taken in working with cultures, as several fatal infections by spores or mycelia have been reported in laboratory workers. Cultures, being puffy or powdery, contaminate the air and workers can be invaded by inhalation. Therefore the plate with the fungus should be placed on a dampened cloth during examination and must be opened carefully.

Reproduction. Fungi are reproduced by the formation of spores, usually by a sexual mechanism (the reproduction of yeasts is asexual only; they multiply by budding). Multiplication of mycelial fungi is mainly apical —at the apex of the hypha.

There are distinguished two main types of spores: ascospores (sexual spores)—they develop from special cells in the mycelium, by nuclear fusion; and thallospores (asexual spores) formed by fermentation of the hypha. They may develop a thick protective wall and are then called chlamydospores. Many other types of spores are designated.

Serologic Characteristics. Some fungi show agglutination or complement-fixation reactions and various phenomena of immunity and hypersensitivity. Recently, serologic typing according to capsular material (carbohydrates, polysaccharides, and proteins) has been used for diagnosis of some
mycoses. A delayed tuberculinlike skin test is diagnostically important in
many mycoses.

Pathogenesis and Pathology. Three important factors must be considered in pathogenesis and pathology of mycoses: endotoxin, multiplication of the fungi (usually very slow), and the phenomenon of hypersensitivity. The mycotic infections are chiefly chronic, varying in severity. They
may be extremely mild; in mycosis of the skin, hair, and nails the fungi are
almost saprophytic and behave as foreign bodies. In some other cases,
mycotic diseases are generalized and even fatal (deep mycosis). Fungi do
not usually produce epidemics. Mycoses are said to be found more frequently in males than in females.

In mycoses, any pathologic process may occur, such as suppuration
(resembling staphylococcal infection) or caseous necrosis with resultant
fibrosis. These may be mistaken for tuberculosis. Some mycoses resemble
cancer. Tubercle-like giant cell granuloma is the most typical finding in
mycosis; in this, the phagocytosis of fungi by reticuloendothelial cells may
remind one of "storage."

Reactions of hypersensitivity occur frequently in mycoses, giving a
valuable diagnostic indication.

Intravenous inoculation of rabbits or intraperitoneal injection of guinea
pigs with fungus culture is often used to determine the pathogenicity of
fungi.

In almost all mycoses, there is a history of injury to the host preceding
invasion by the fungus.

Polymorphism is a typical feature of fungi. Their morphologic and
biologic characteristics are not constant; hence the classification is complex
and confusing. In medical practice, the most convenient division of fungi
is based on anatomic location of the mycotic lesions. Two groups are distinguished: deep mycosis, chiefly with systemic involvement, and superficial mycosis, extremely rarely affecting the general health. The eye is
involved usually secondarily to systemic mycosis, by continuation from
surrounding areas, or by metastasis from distant organs. Both secondary
and primary ocular mycoses, although rare in the past, are now increasing.
The importance of mycoses in ophthalmology will be briefly described.

REFERENCES

1. Aldridge, J. S., and Kirk, R.   Mycetoma of the eyelid, Brit. J. Ophth., 24:211, 1940.
2. Anderson, B., Roberts, S. S., Jr., Gonzalez, C., and Chick, E. W.   Mycotic ulcerative keratitis, Arch. Ophth., 62:169, 1959.
3. Birge, H. L.   Ocular aspects of mycotic infection, Arch. Ophth., 47:354, 1952.

4. Breed, R. S., et al. Bergey's Manual of Determinative Bacteriology, 7th ed., Baltimore, Williams & Wilkins Co., 1957.
5. Conant, N. F., Smith, D. T., Baker, R. D., Callaway, J. L., and Martin, D. S. Manual of Clinical Mycology, 2nd ed., Philadelphia and London, W. B. Saunders Co., 1958.
6. Dubos, R. J. Bacterial and Mycotic Infections of Man, 3rd ed., Philadelphia, J. B. Lippincott Co., 1958.
7. Duke-Elder, W. S. Text-book of Ophthalmology, St. Louis, C. V. Mosby Co., 1946, vol. 2.
8. Fazakas, S. Comprehensive report on secondary mycoses in diseases of the palpebral margin, the conjunctiva and the cornea, Surv. Ophth., 5:419, 1960.
9. Fine, B. S., and Zimmerman, L. E. Exogenous intraocular fungus infections, Am. J. Ophth., 48:151, 1959.
10. Hammeke, J. C., and Ellis, P. P. Mycotic flora of the conjunctiva, Am. J. Ophth., 49:1174, 1960.
11. Levitt, J. M. Ocular manifestations of coccidioidomycosis, Am. J. Ophth., 31:1626, 1948.
12. Ley, A. P., and Sanders, T. E. Fungus keratitis, Arch. Ophth., 56:257, 1956.
13. Mitsui, Y., and Hanabusa, J. Corneal infections after cortisone therapy, Brit. J. Ophth., 39:244, 1955.
14. Rychener, R. O. Intra-ocular mycosis, Tr. Am. Ophth. Soc., 31:477, 1933.
15. Simon, F. A. Allergic conjunctivitis due to fungi, J.A.M.A., 110:440, 1938.
16. Smith, D. T., and Conant, N. F. Zinsser Microbiology, 12th ed., New York, Appleton-Century-Crofts, Inc., 1960.

ACTINOMYCETACEAE

Actinomycetaceae were once regarded as true fungi. Now many consider them filamentous bacteria; others, as midway between fungi and bacteria. Therefore, confusion arises, and further clarification of their classification is needed.

The family *Actinomycetaceae* includes the genera *Actinomyces* and *Nocardia;* both are important in human pathology. The genus *Actinomyces* is mainly composed of anaerobic obligate parasites, and *Nocardia* of aerobic facultative parasites, although oxygen requirements vary in the same genus.

ACTINOMYCES

Actinomyces species cause actinomycosis; the species *A. bovis* infects cattle, and the species *A. israelii* affects man, but some regard them as the same species. However, saprophytic species of *Actinomyces* predominate, being found on grain, grass, or water. Many varieties, including pathogenic ones, are present in the human teeth, tonsils, or pharynx.

Morphology. These organisms are long filaments or rods with clubbed ends. They stain gram-positive (nonacid-fast), resembling corynebacteria in their irregular staining, arrangement, and club shape. Some filaments have false branching, true branching being uncommon. Later, the filaments undergo segmentation into rods which are often clubbed or into coccoid bodies which are regarded as spores.

Culture.   Species of *Actinomyces* grow anaerobically and slowly, taking two weeks or more. Blood dextrose agar in shake culture may be used. Sabouraud's agar will not support these organisms. The colonies are small, irregular, grayish or white, and their rough surface appears nodular. Most strains are nonhemolytic and nonproteolytic. In smears from a colony, long branching filaments are seen.

Staphylococci are usually present in the culture as secondary invaders.

Pathology.   Actinomycosis may be localized or generalized, and it tends toward chronicity. The process, often preceded by trauma, involves mainly the face or neck, less often the lungs or abdomen. Nodules, with central caseation surrounded by granulomatous tissue, are typical; they frequently become abscessed. Tissue sections under the microscope show small, round, yellow granules called drüsen, each of which consists of a mass of branching filaments. They are the best material for laboratory diagnosis. Because of their color, drüsen are sometimes rather confusingly designated sulfur granules. The periphery of a drüsen is surrounded by radiating clubs, whence originated the now seldom-used term, ray fungus, for actinomyces.

Hypersensitivity to actinomyces is a frequent phenomenon.

Findings in the Eye.   Involvement of the eyelids, though infrequent, usually occurs by contiguous spread from adjacent parts of the face or sinuses. The infection is occasionally primary. Indolent subcutaneous nodules develop; usually multiple, they become interconnected, causing a honeycomb appearance. Spreading to the surface of the skin, the nodules break down, and a purulent discharge follows, which contains yellowish or greenish granules (drüsen).

Actinomycosis may also involve the lid margins, causing many small, indolent abscesses with a tendency to ulcerate.

An exudative, purulent conjunctivitis may occur, particularly in children. The painless and freely movable nodules sometimes occur on the bulbar conjunctiva, near the limbus. Their association with blepharoconjunctivitis has been observed. Intraocular infection following cataract extraction, uveitis, or corneal ulcers of varying severity, and infection of the orbit from surrounding infected sinuses have been reported.

Painless nodules or abscesses in deep tissue often result in fistulae, and the presence of drüsen is characteristic. The clinical picture is not always pathognomonic, and microscopic diagnosis, particularly of the granules, is most important.

Streptothrix

The historic background of *Streptothrix* has been given by Pine et al. More than 100 years have passed since von Graefe established the fungus etiology of the concretions in the lacrimal canal. The species of fungus was not identified. The name *Streptothrix* was given in 1875 by Cohn. Since the condition is rare and cultivation of the organism is not available, its identification is not yet established. The name *Streptothrix* has usually been used on the basis of clinical features, being almost pathognomonic for concretions in the canaliculus. Recently, various species (*Candida, Nocardia, Actinomyces*) have been identified as causes of lacrimal concretions. Therefore the question persists concerning the identification of *Streptothrix*.

Several investigators established *Streptothrix* as anaerobic *Actinomyces*. However, even recently the term was used as a synonym for both aerobic and anaerobic *Actinomyces*. The classification remains to be fully clarified, as well as that of the family *Actinomycetaceae* itself. Some general bacteriologists propose that the name *Streptothrix* be abandoned. However, in ophthalmology this name is widely accepted. There appears to be small reason to discard it even in the future when the genus is fully established. The name *Streptothrix* can be saved as an ophthalmic species of this genus. It seems advisable for clinicians to use the term "concretions of the canaliculi" or "canaliculitis" instead of streptothricosis. Identification of the organism is important for further clarification of nomenclature.

Morphology.   *Streptothrix* is studied in material obtained from the concretions of canaliculitis. The concretion must be squeezed and crushed on a slide; saline solution is added to this very dry material, then the preparation is gram stained. In our laboratory we found that Giemsa staining reveals the structure more distinctly. The organisms are branched filaments which readily segment into rods and coccoid forms. Staining by the gram stain varies. Some bacillary forms are gram-negative. According to Ellis, the gram-positive coccoid forms, which he calls "streptococci," are actually arthrospores or oidiospores. Because of the polymorphic appearance in smears, *Streptothrix* can easily be confused with bacteria. Besides, bacterial secondary invaders are always present in the concretions. All this must be thoroughly considered, since diagnosis is usually determined by microscopic examination of original smears.

Cultivation.   The cultivation of *Streptothrix* is difficult because the organism is anaerobic, and the concretions usually contain numerous secondary bacterial invaders. However, the organisms are successfully cultivated in Brewer's medium, in an anaerobic zone of the tube. It requires about nine days. The growth consists mainly of a mass of hyphae, chains of cocci, and bacilli.

Findings in the Eye.   *Streptothrix* is the almost exclusive etiologic agent of mycotic canaliculitis. Other ocular manifestations of *Streptothrix* mycosis are rare.

MYCOTIC CANALICULITIS.   This infection is practically restricted to women. It is usually unilateral, the lower canaliculus being chiefly involved. Initially, lacrimation is the only symptom and the process can be easily overlooked. Later, a characteristic localized swelling develops in the area of the canaliculus. An accumulation of concretions causes the swelling, but local inflammation is mild. The related punctum lacrimalis becomes dilated, and later a chronic, stubborn unilateral conjunctivitis, sometimes with copious yellowish or greenish discharge, occurs.

The concretions needed for diagnostic examination should be expressed by careful squeezing. Put any suitable hard support behind the canaliculus and press. Sometimes the canaliculus has to be split to obtain the concretions. According to their age, the color varies from gray to yellow to brown. Microscopically, a concretion consists of a mass of branching filaments, spores, and varying bacteria (Plate XXX, 2).

Treatment. This requires complete removal of the concretions. Curettage is the simplest method; this is usually preceded by splitting the canaliculus through the punctum. The procedure must be done thoroughly, but gently, to prevent recurrence and spreading of the infection. The treatment is completed by instillation of a 1 per cent solution of tincture of iodine or a solution of penicillin.

Leptothrix

According to Bergey's classification, *Leptothrix* is the name applied to the algae commonly found in ponds. These are nonbranching and ensheathed filamentous bacteria, nonpathogenic and unrelated to the genus *Actinomyces*.

However in ophthalmology, *Leptothrix* is of special interest as a cause of conjunctivoglandular Parinaud's syndrome. The condition was first described by Verhoeff in 1918. Using a special staining technic, he demonstrated the organisms in a section of tissue involved. Later, the organism was cultured by Verhoeff and King, Wright, Ridley and Smith, and Gifford and Alexander, either from biopsy or from the pus of the regional glands. The organisms have usually been considered a species of the genus *Actinomyces*. All this study is insufficient. The name is confusing, and more culture study is needed for identification.

Morphology. *Leptothrix* is described in ophthalmology as morphologically similar to *Streptothrix*, except that it is usually unbranched (Plate XXX, 5). To demonstrate *Leptothrix* in section is not easy, and the material has to be obtained from essential lesions, fixed in Zenker's fluid, and stained by Verhoeff's modified gram method. The section reveals granules and threads, the granules being gram-positive and sometimes arranged in chains. Some filaments are gram-positive, others gram-negative.

Cultivation is difficult and is seldom used. Positive cultivation on serum-glucose medium and on Brewer's medium has been recorded.

Findings in the Eye. Leptothricosis of the eye is rare and is almost exclusively found in children and young adults, chiefly males. The disease appears more commonly in winter. Rabbits, horses, and particularly cats may act as reservoirs for this organism.

The conjunctiva is the only known site of invasion, which is usually preceded by trauma. The incubation period is three to seven days. Leptothricosis of the conjunctiva is characterized by nodules—single or more frequently multiple. These are sometimes pinpoint and scattered on the palpebral conjunctiva; they are grayish or yellowish. Large, mushroom-shaped lesions may occur. Follicles are usually present.

The bulbar conjunctiva, near the limbus, is most often affected. The lesions have no tendency to ulcerate, and the cornea is uninvolved. The lids are usually markedly swollen, and enlargement of the preauricular and submaxillary glands (oculoglandular Parinaud's syndrome) is constantly associated with the condition.

Catarrhal conjunctivitis of the angular or membranous types may also occur.

Treatment. Iodide or sulfonamides are used systemically. Complete incision of the involved area is indicated. However, even after surgery, the conjunctivitis as well as enlargement of the preauricular glands may persist for a long time.

NOCARDIA

Nocardia has recently been regarded as an aerobic genus of the family *Actinomycetaceae*. The genus includes many species living free in nature. *Nocardia asteroides* has been found to be a human pathogen.

Morphology. *Nocardia* shows branching filaments, some of which have a tendency to fragment into rods and cocci (Plate XXX, 4). All of the species stain gram-positive. Some are also acid-fast and may be mistaken for the tubercle bacillus.

Yellowish, red, or brown mycelial granules, consisting of the organisms, may be seen in the pus. This is the best specimen for laboratory examination.

Culture. *Nocardia* grows readily on a variety of simple media, at room temperature. Sabouraud's medium is usually used; on this, growth takes three to four weeks. On simple media the growth is even slower. The colonies are wrinkled and crumbling, resembling those of mycobacteria (Plate XXX, 3). However, a great variation of appearance of the cultures, even on the same medium, is typical. Some colonies produce aerial mycelia; these have a chalky and powdery appearance. The color of the colonies may differ, being creamy, yellow, pink, or red.

Pathology. Nocardiosis is a chronic, suppurative process associated with granuloma (mycetoma) and draining sinuses. The pus usually contains granules consisting of *Nocardia* organisms. The process is found chiefly in bones, and is characterized by multiple lesions followed by drainage. After months or even years, deformities particularly of the foot (madura foot) ensue. *Nocardia* contaminates wounds, causing localized mycetoma. When inhaled, the organism may cause pulmonary disease, usually manifested as tuberculosis-like infection. A similar process may occur in the brain.

Nocardiosis may remain localized or become generalized by metastasis.

Findings in the Eye. Little has been published about ocular nocardiosis. Chronic keratoconjunctivitis may occur secondarily to nocardiosis of adjacent areas. Patches of granulation occur on the lower lid, followed by scarring. Schardt has described a case of large, dirty corneal ulceration with overhanging edge, of chronic duration. *Nocardia asteroides* infection of the lacrimal duct has been reported by Penikett and Rees.

REFERENCES

1. Benedict, W. L., and Iverson, H. A. Chronic keratoconjunctivitis associated with nocardia, Arch. Ophth., 32:89, 1944.
2. Breed, R. S., and Conn, H. J. The nomenclature of the *Actinomycetaceae*, J. Bact., 4:585, 1919.
3. Bruce, G. M., and Locatcher-Khorazo, D. Actinomyces: recovery of the streptothrix in a case of superficial punctate keratitis, Arch. Ophth., 27:294, 1942.
4. Donahue, H. C. Unusual mycotic infection of the lacrimal canaliculi and conjunctiva, Am. J. Ophth., 32:207, 1949.
5. Elliot, A. J. Streptothricosis of the lacrimal canaliculi, Am. J. Ophth., 24:682, 1941.
6. Ellis, P. P., Bausor, S. C., and Fulmer, J. M. Streptothrix canaliculitis, Am. J. Ophth., 52:36, 1961.
7. Gibson, J. M. Actinomycosis of the canaliculi with invasion of tissue in one case, Brit. J. Ophth., 36:522, 1952.
8. Gifford, S. R., and Day, A. A. Leptotrichosis conjunctivae, Arch. Ophth., 31:423, 1944.
9. Gordon, R. E., and Smith, M. M. Proposed group of characters for the separation of streptomyces and nocardia, J. Bact., 69:147, 1955.
10. Hagedoorn, A. Concretions in a lacrimal canaliculus caused by actinomyces, Arch. Ophth., 23:689, 1940.
11. Henry, M. Oculoglandular conjunctivitis due to leptothrix (Abstract), Am. J. Ophth., 34:138, 1951.
12. Kant, A. Unusual case of leptothricosis conjunctivae, Am. J. Ophth., 31:607, 1948.
13. Lemoine, A. N. Parinaud's conjunctivitis, with demonstration of the leptothrix of Verhoeff, J.A.M.A., 82:537, 1924.
14. Nagel, C. S. G. Fungus concretion in lacrimal canaliculus (streptothricosis, actinomycosis), Am. J. Ophth., 3:327, 1920.
15. Penikett, E. J. K., and Rees, D. L. *Nocardia asteroides* infection, Am. J. Ophth., 53:1006, 1962.
16. Pine, L., and Hardin, H. *Actinomyces israelii*: a cause of lacrimal canaliculitis in man, J. Bact., 78:164, 1959.
17. —————— Hardin, H., Turner, L., and Roberts, S. S. Actinomycotic lacrimal canaliculitis, Am. J. Ophth., 49:1278, 1960.
18. Ridley, F., and Smith, C. Leptotrichosis conjunctivae, Brit. J. Ophth., 36:328, 1952.
19. Sanford, A. H., and Voelker, M. Actinomycosis in the United States, Arch. Surg., 11:809, 1925.
20. Schardt, W. M., Unsworth, A. C., and Hayes, C. V. Corneal ulcer due to *Nocardia asteroides*, Am. J. Ophth., 42:303, 1956.
21. Smith, C. H. Ocular actinomycosis, Proc. Roy. Soc. Med., 46:209, 1953.
22. Theodore, F. H. Streptothrix as a cause of follicular conjunctivitis and other obscure conjunctivitides, Am. J. Ophth., 33:1225, 1950.
23. Thorson, J. A., and Mueller, E. F. Probable actinomycosis of the orbit, J. Iowa M. Soc., 31:70, 1941.
24. Verhoeff, F. H. Observations on Parinaud's conjunctivitis (leptothricosis conjunctivae), Am. J. Ophth., 1:705, 1918.
25. Wright, R. E. Isolation of Verhoeff's leptothrix in a case of Parinaud's syndrome, Arch. Ophth., 18:233, 1937.

DEEP MYCOSES

Unlike the superficial mycoses which are usually localized, the deep ones may become systemic or even fatal. Yeastlike fungi are responsible for most of the deep mycoses.

Candida

Many synonyms exist for this large group, among which *Monilia* was the most popular. Now the name *Candida*, proposed by Berkhout, is generally accepted. *Candida albicans* is thought to be the only pathogenic strain. This is a yeastlike fungus which grows best in environments with a high sugar content, especially fruits. Growth is poor in soil. The fungus has been demonstrated in the normal human flora on mucous membranes of the eye and in the respiratory, gastrointestinal, and female genital tracts. It has also been identified as part of the normal flora in a variety of animals.

The disease candidiasis is most common among dishwashers, whose hands must remain moist, and among fruit packers.

Overuse of antibiotics and steroids, with consequent disturbance of the normal flora, is believed responsible for the recent increased incidence of candidiasis. The tetracyclines may even stimulate the growth of candida. Pregnancy, alcoholism, vascular stress, or heavy sweating are predisposing factors.

Morphology. *Candida albicans* has a typical yeast morphology, showing a small, ovoid, or cylindric cell four or five times as big as that of staphylococci. The larger size of the individual cells, their budding, and more dense gram-positive staining are important practical criteria in distinguishing candida cells from cocci in the smear. Many of the cells have heavy cell walls which possibly are composed of cellulose. The cells are most often arranged in irregular, clusterlike masses (Plate XXXII, 1). Atypical chains or filaments resembling mycelia are sometimes seen.

Culture. *Candida* species grow on all ordinary media both at room temperature and at 37° C. Sabouraud's glucose agar is preferable, as growth is faster on it, requiring only three to five days. Blood agar may be used. The colonies are typically cream-colored, small, round, opaque, dry or moist, and resemble staphylococcal colonies (Plate XXXII, 2, 3). They produce pseudomycelia and have a distinct yeastlike odor.

Corn-meal agar is used to stimulate the production of chlamydospores, characteristic for the pathogenic strain.

Pathogenicity and Pathology. Rabbits are particularly susceptible to *Candida albicans* and are used to prove pathogenicity. Intravenous injection with 1 ml of 1 per cent saline suspension of *C. albicans* infects rabbits and causes death in four to five days. The kidney abscess is characteristic pathology.

Candidiasis is a localized disease which rarely metastasizes. When it does, it may be fatal. Ocular candidiasis is increasingly reported.

The diseases caused by *C. albicans* are thrushlike infections. They usually develop in newborn children, infected from a mother having vulvovaginitis. Elderly persons, especially if debilitated, are apt to be affected. In generalized cases, the most usual developments are severe lung infection, meningitis, or endocarditis.

Characteristics of the tissue involved and the degree of hypersensitivity to the fungus are the chief factors determining the pathologic picture. The eczematous process, vesicular or pustulous, is typical for the skin infection; infected mucous membranes have a pseudomembrane, giving a patchy appearance; and for the inner organs, the granulomatous process is characteristic. The granuloma is similar to tuberculous granuloma, with giant epithelial cells, necrosis, and central abscess formation. The fungi are usually found in this necrotic area.

Findings in the Eye.   Unfortunately, there is no consistency of nomenclature in clinical reports; the term "monilia" is still frequently used. Any structure of the eye and its adnexa may be affected by candida, either primarily or secondarily. Although ocular candidiasis is infrequent and uncommon, it now appears to be increasing. Lesions of the lid skin are usually associated with generalized candidiasis of the face. These are grayish or reddish, scaly, and definitely marginated. Simultaneously, vesicles, pustules, or scaly, red, sharply marginated lesions are found at the lid margins. Eczematous blepharitis or angular blepharoconjunctivitis has also been observed. Patchy necrotic blepharitis in infants, associated with generalized candidiasis, has been reported.

CONJUNCTIVITIS.   A pseudomembranous, diffuse or localized necrotic conjunctivitis is found in association with similar manifestations of other mucosa. A stringy, mucopurulent discharge is commonly present. Lesions of a granulomatous nature may also occur. Norton described thrush of the conjunctiva appearing as four white patches or scabs, symmetrically placed outside the cornea in the palpebral fissure. They were easily removed. The process was indolent, without reaction of the conjunctiva. The condition may be confused with Bitot's spots, and examination of scrapings is essential.

KERATITIS.   The manifestations of candida keratitis are varied. Peculiar round, shallow, indolent, gray, and dry corneal ulcers with undermined edges may develop. Near the limbus, the lesions may resemble fascicular keratitis. Central serpiginous hypopyon ulcer resembling a bacterial ulcer may also be caused by candida. A deep ulcer showing a dry necrotic mass resembling bread crumbs, with a pink, glistening base, may result in perforation and panophthalmitis. This is easily mistaken for a tuberculous infection. A type of dendritic keratitis associated with a foreign body was reported by Sykes. The ulcer was covered by a gray adherent membrane in which candida was revealed.

We have observed two cases of keratitis caused by *Candida albicans*. One occurred in generalized candidiasis. Several yellowish infiltrates, sharply marginated, were present. These were also a few small ulcers, covered by masses resembling bread crumbs (Plate XXXI, 1). Fluorescein staining was negative. Numerous yeastlike bodies and filamentous forms were found in direct scrapings (Plate XXXI, 5). *C. albicans* was identified by cultures, and pathogenicity was proven by injection into a rabbit. The second patient developed a hypopyon ulcerative keratitis after prolonged used of antibiotics. The process was localized and responded to treatment (Plate XXXI, 2, 4).

Infection of the orbit, uveitis, or dacryocystitis may occasionally develop by continuation from adjacent tissue.

Diagnosis. *C. albicans* is often found in man, either in normal flora or as a secondary invader. Hence it is difficult to prove candida as a primary etiologic agent. Direct examination of fresh material from the lesion is the most important for diagnosis. One drop of 10 per cent potassium hydroxide is added to the exudate, which is then examined in fresh preparation after gentle heating of the slide to clear the exudate.

Staining of the scraping by the gram stain is valuable. Culture and demonstration of chlamydospores are diagnostically important. To demonstrate chlamydospores, direct examination of fresh culture on corn-meal agar is used. Place the plate on the stage, cover the peripheral zone of the growth with a coverglass, and examine under the low-power objective. The chlamydospores appear as thick-walled, terminal cells, being the resting spores of pseudohyphae (Plate XXXII, 4).

Skin testing may have value for diagnosis. It is needed to determine and evaluate possible hypersensitivity to the fungus.

Treatment. Patients with systemic candidiasis or those with hypersensitivity to this fungus present a difficult therapeutic problem.

The localized process may be treated surgically and topically with good results. For topical treatment, any alkaline lotion for the eye may be used. When the disease is external, gentian violet (1 per cent solution in 70 per cent alcohol) is recommended for painting the skin, including lid margins. Cauterization of the cornea with tincture of iodine is sometimes effective. In addition, potassium iodide may be given by mouth, provided a skin test is negative for candida hypersensitivity. In hypersensitive patients, potassium iodide may cause dissemination of the disease process. The iodide is usually given by slow method—starting with 3 drops three times a day, 1 drop is added daily to each dose until 20 drops per dose is reached. The treatment is discontinued in reverse fashion.

Treatment has to be stopped if iodism develops. A low carbohydrate diet is recommended. X-ray therapy may be useful.

Nystatin (Mycostatin) and Mycosteclin are usually combined with any of the above mentioned therapies.

Blastomyces dermatitidis

Blastomycosis is clinically manifested in three forms: cutaneous, pulmonary, or systemic. The process is usually granulomatous, similar clinically and histologically to tuberculosis. The name North American blastomycosis is used. It is also known as Gilchrist's disease, after the investigator who first described the fungus, *Blastomyces dermatitidis*, in 1896.

Morphology. The fungus appears in tissue or exudate as a large, spherical, thick-walled, double-contoured, budding, yeastlike body. The organism is smaller in tissue, and may be mistaken for *Histoplasma capsulatum*. On the culture medium, the fungus first appears in the form of yeastlike bodies, which soon become moldlike filaments (Plate XXXIII, 4).

Culture. The fungus grows readily on Sabouraud's medium at room temperature. At first, the colonies are smooth and yeastlike, resembling staphylococci, but hyphal aerial projections quickly develop. The colonies are initially white and cottony (Plate XXXIII, 2), but later become brownish and prickly. In smear from the colonies, filamentous forms predominate. The filaments, when subcultured, again become yeastlike bodies.

The fungus also grows on blood agar, but more slowly, developing wrinkled, waxy colonies; in smear, budding cells predominate.

Pathology. Blastomycosis of the skin is a chronic disease which, if untreated, may last for years. The lesions are either papulopustulous or granulomatous and usually result in regional adenopathy. The granuloma frequently turns into an abscess which is typically surrounded by disseminated, tiny abscesses. The papulopustular lesions generally become ulcerated. Their base is papillary or verrucose and is covered by a dirty pink exudate. The papillary hypertrophy may resemble carcinoma.

The process may become generalized by metastasis to the eye, the lungs or other internal organs, or the bones. The systemic disease is very serious, sometimes fatal.

Findings in the Eye. Blastomycosis of the eye is relatively uncommon. It has a predilection for the lids, appearing in the form of small abscesses around the lashes. According to Wood, the lids may be involved in one fourth of all cases. The process is destructive and is followed by ectropion and scarring. Blastomycosis of the conjunctiva or cornea is usually secondary to blepharitis. Spreading of the mycosis from the lid margin over the entire face in unrecognized cases has been reported. An opinion exists that the conjunctiva is immune to *Blastomyces dermatitidis*, since the process may spread from the lid directly to the cornea, avoiding the conjunctiva. However, blastomycosis of the conjunctiva has been diagnosed by Theodorides; the conjunctivitis was characterized by small, whitish spots (resembling Bitot's spots) on the bulbar conjunctiva of the open area. In this case, the identification of blastomycosis cannot be regarded as fully confirmed, since the culture was negative and the diagnosis was made in smear only.

The keratitis is rare and usually ulcerative, similar to candida ulcers.

Blockage of the nasolacrimal duct by a mycotic mass, resulting in the development of diverticular dacryocystitis, may occur.

Metastatic uveitis in systemic blastomycosis is not as rare as has generally been supposed (Cassady). Metastatic retinal or optic nerve mycoses are unusual manifestations described. Papilledema (Plate XXXIII, 1) associated with systemic blastomycosis may occur.

Diagnosis. The roof of the lesion must be removed to obtain pus for examination, and the fresh untreated material examined directly. This is mounted on a slide in a drop of 10 per cent potassium hydroxide, a coverglass is added, and the slide is gently heated to clear the specimen. The preparation is then examined under subdued light. The thick walls of the budding bodies have a double-contoured appearance characteristic of blastomyces (Plate XXXIII, 3).

The blastomycin skin test may be valuable, though it can sometimes be positive in healthy persons.

Treatment. If the process is local, excision of the lesion should be performed. Radiation therapy may be useful early in the infection.

The treatment of generalized blastomycosis is a much more difficult problem. Iodides, radiation, or desensitization may be employed. Vaccination is valuable when hypersensitivity exists. Before vaccination, preliminary testing by intracutaneous injection in a dose of 0.1 ml should be performed, then the vaccine diluted according to the size of the skin reaction. Vaccination is highly recommended before starting the iodine treatment, since dissemination of the mycosis may follow iodine therapy.

Stilbamidine or Propamidine may be effective.

Histoplasma capsulatum

Histoplasmosis has been recognized clinically in the past few years. A pure culture of the fungus was obtained only in 1934 by De Monbreun.

Histoplasma capsulatum is a yeastlike fungus causing histoplasmosis with varied clinical manifestations. It is a highly infectious mycosis usually appearing as a primary pulmonary disease. Its intracellular nature in the reticuloendothelial system and healing by calcification are characteristics similar to those of toxoplasma.

Meleney, reviewing the literature in 1940, found 32 cases of histoplasmosis, with no ocular involvement reported. However, the incidence varies geographically. It is endemic in the Central Mississippi and Ohio valleys, in Oklahoma, and other localities. Incidence is low in Europe and Central America, but high in Mexico and Panama.

Histoplasma capsulatum may infect many animals—dogs, cats, rodents, or others. The infection is transmitted through biting insects, or by animals.

Morphology. *H. capsulatum* is a budding, oval, yeastlike organism usually found within endothelial, mononuclear, or polymorphonuclear cells.

The intracellular organisms appear as small, oval bodies resembling protozoa (Plate XXXIII, 5). The fungus can be demonstrated in exudate, blood smear, or tissue section, stained with Giemsa or Wright stain, and examined with the oil immersion objective. Typical yeastlike budding bodies or tuberculate spores are found in fresh preparation from the culture.

Culture. *H. capsulatum* can be cultured on all common laboratory media. On Sabouraud's medium, it grows at room temperature, taking about one month. Initially the growth is cottony and white, becoming brown in older culture (Plate XXXIII, 6). On blood agar, the growth resembles staphylococci, but a mycelial growth may also occur (Plate XXXIII, 7).

Pathology. Histoplasmosis is most often found as a primary pulmonary infection, which heals by multiple areas of calcification. It may frequently be manifested as an ulceration of the nasopharyngeal cavities or of the intestine. Generalized adenopathy and secondary anemia or leukopenia usually accompanies the process. Laboratory personnel working with the fungus have been infected. The disease is often asymptomatic, and the patient develops sensitivity to histoplasmin about one week after the initial infection.

Findings in the Eye. Histoplasmosis of the eye is reported extremely rarely. However, the conjunctiva can be involved in association with other mucosa; histoplasmosis has been suggested in generalized adenopathy. A case with a tumorlike ulceration of the palpebral conjunctiva has been recorded.

Diagnosis. Determination of the diagnosis is based on finding intracellular yeastlike fungi in peripheral blood smears or other specimens. However, the culture is more important for diagnosis by typical colonies and particularly by tuberculate spores characteristic of *H. capsulatum*. This is demonstrated in wet preparation mounted in cotton blue solution. The typical spherical thick-walled spores have fingerlike projections (Plate XXXIII, 8).

Treatment. Surgical treatment is indicated for localized histoplasmosis. The generalized process presents a problem, as there is no specific treatment. Iodides, heavy metals, penicillin, or streptomycin may be useful.

Cryptococcus neoformans
(*Torula histolytica*)

Cryptococcus is a yeastlike fungus, nonsporulating and nonmycelial. The species *Cryptococcus neoformans* is pathogenic for man. Soil, milk, and especially pigeons' nests are considered the most common sources of infection.

C. neoformans may involve any part of the body, but has a predilection for the central nervous system. Chronic meningitis is a typical manifestation of cryptococcosis; the ocular nervous tissue is often secondarily involved.

Morphology. Cryptococci are large, thick-walled, budding bodies, round or elongated. These are usually arranged in a honeycomb-appearing mass (Plate XXXIV, 5). The organism is surrounded by a thick, gelatinous capsule, usually twice as wide as the cell body. The capsule is best demonstrated with India ink, in fresh preparation.

Culture. The fungus grows on Sabouraud's medium, slowly and at room temperature. Colonies appear white, wrinkled, and granular. Later, they become moist and shiny, have a tendency to coalesce, and are tan to brown in color (Plate XXXIV, 3). Budding cells are found and a capsule is readily demonstrated at this stage. There is no spore formation. On blood agar, the colonies are gray, opaque, round, and glistening, resembling staphylococci (Plate XXXIV, 4).

Pathology. Primary lesions are mainly found in the lungs, rarely on the skin or mucosa, and are associated with adenopathy. The organisms may spread to the brain, causing chronic meningitis lasting many years and resembling a brain tumor. The signs are the same as in any other meningitis, but despite the severity of the symptoms, acute inflammation is usually absent.

Human transmission of the mycosis is unknown.

Findings in the Eye. The eye is rarely involved, usually secondarily to meningitis. Ocular symptoms of the meningitis are: amblyopia, strabismus, nystagmus, ptosis, and diplopia. Neuroretinitis, choked disc, and cystoid degeneration or hemorrhages of the retina have been observed. The only case of intraocular cryptococcosis has been described by Weiss et al.[27] This appeared as a binocular cystic growth in the retina, from which *Cryptococcus neoformans* was isolated. Orbital cryptococcosis has been reported. The fungus has also been found by Cohen in association with Hodgkin's disease.[6] The eyebrow can be the site of a primary lesion (Plate XXXIV, 1).

Diagnosis of cryptococcic mycosis is difficult for the ophthalmologist and is usually made post mortem. (For exception, see Weiss.)

Diagnosis. This is determined by finding *Cryptococcus neoformans*, either in the specimen or in the culture. The material may be obtained by aspiration, swabbing, or scraping the tissue from the biopsy specimen. Mount the material in a drop of diluted India ink and examine it under a coverglass while the preparation is wet; avoid drying. India ink is used for contrast with the capsule. The wide capsule is important for differential diagnosis (Plate XXXIV, 2). The frozen section of tissue is mounted in undiluted Giemsa stain. The periodic acid-Schiff technic also gives an excellent result. The fungus in section is found free or within giant cells. To prove the pathogenicity of the organisms, a cultural suspension is injected into mice, intraperitoneally, intracerebrally, or intravenously.

Virulence of the strain is indicated by meningitis or death of the mice.

Treatment. Actidione and amphotericin B have been recommended. Intravenous amphotericin B (30 mg daily) is effective in the disseminated process. Good results have been recorded with intravenous Mycostatin. The addition of sulfonamides to the above treatments may be helpful.

REFERENCES

1. Beamer, P. R., Smith, E. B., and Barnett, H. L.   Histoplasmosis: report of case in infant and experimental observations, J. Pediat., 24:270, 1944.
2. Birge, H. L.   The diagnosis of ocular mycotic infections, Arch. Ophth., 46:225, 1951.
3. Broders, A. C., Dochat, G. R., Herrell, W. E., and Vaughn, L. D.   An unusual case of histoplasmosis, Proc. Staff Meet. Mayo Clin., 19:123, 1944.
4. Campbell, R. M., and Parrot, M. H.   Vulvovaginal moniliasis, Am. J. Obst. & Gynec., 59:1005, 1950.
5. Cassady, J. V.   Uveal blastomycosis, Arch. Ophth., 35:84, 1946.
6. Cohen, M.   Binocular papilledema in a case of torulosis associated with Hodgkin's disease, Arch. Ophth., 32:477, 1944.
7. Day, R.   Experimental ocular histoplasmosis, Am. J. Ophth., 32:1317, 1949.
8. De Monbreun, W. A.   The cultivation and cultural characteristics of Darling's *Histoplasma capsulatum*, Am. J. Trop. Med., 14:93, 1934.
9. Ferguson, A. S.   Blastomycosis of eye and face secondary to lung infection, Brit. M. J., 1:442, 1928.
10. Fine, M., and Waring, W. S.   Mycotic obstruction of the nasolacrimal duct (*Candida albicans*), Arch. Ophth., 38:39, 1947.
11. Gifford, S. R.   Diseases of the eye and adnexa due to fungi and the higher bacteria, Arch. Ophth., 57:224, 1928.
12. Krause, A. C., and Hopkins, W. G.   Ocular manifestation of histoplasmosis, Am. J. Ophth., 34:564, 1951.
13. Maddren, R. F.   Monilial conjunctivitis, Am. J. Ophth., 24:1307, 1941.
14. Manchester, P. T., Jr., and Georg, L. K.   Corneal ulcer due to *Candida parapsilosis* (*C. parakrusei*), J.A.M.A., 171:1339, 1959.
15. McKee, S. H.   Blastomycoses of the cornea, Intern. Clin., 3:50, 1926.
16. Meleney, H. E.   Histoplasmosis (reticulo-endothelial cytomycosis), Am. J. Trop. Med., 20:603, 1940.
17. Mendelblatt, D. L.   Moniliasis, Am. J. Ophth., 36:379, 1953.
18. Mitsui, Y., and Hanabusa, J.   Corneal infections after cortisone therapy, Brit. J. Ophth., 39:244, 1955.
19. Newton, J. C., and Tulevech, C. B.   Lacrimal canaliculitis due to *Candida albicans*, Am. J. Ophth., 53:933, 1962.
20. Norton, A. H.   Thrush of the conjunctiva, Am. J. Ophth., 10:357, 1927.
21. Riley, W. A., and Watson, C. J.   Histoplasmosis of Darling with report of a case originating in Minnesota, Am. J. Trop. Med., 6:271, 1926.
22. Schwartz, V. J.   Intra-ocular blastomycosis, Arch. Ophth., 5:581, 1931.
23. Smith, J. L., and Jones, D. B.   Experimental avian ocular histoplasmosis, Arch. Ophth., 67:349, 1962.
24. Sykes, E. M.   Fungus infection of the cornea: case report of keratomycosis due to Monilia, Texas J. Med., 42:330, 1946.
25. Theodorides, E., and Koutrolikos, D.   Blastomycosis of the conjunctiva, Am. J. Ophth., 36:978, 1953.
26. Van Buren, J. M.   Septic retinitis due to *Candida albicans* (Abstract), Am. J. Ophth., 46:277, 1958.
27. Weiss, C., Perry, I. H., and Shevky, M. C.   Infection of the human eye with *Cryptococcus neoformans* (*Torula histolytica; Cryptococcus hominis*), Arch. Ophth., 39:739, 1948.
28. Wilder, W. H.   Blastomycosis of the eyelid, J.A.M.A., 43:2026, 1904.
29. Wood, C. A.   Blastomycosis of the ocular structures, especially of the eyelids, Ann. Ophth., 13:92, 1904.
30. Woods, A. C., and Wahlen, H. E.   The probable role of benign histoplasmosis in the etiology of granulomatous uveitis, Am. J. Ophth., 49:205, 1960.

Plates XXX–XXXIV

PLATE XXX

1. Mycotic canaliculitis shown in rare locale (upper canaliculus). The surrounding area is swollen but not inflamed; white spot is an exudate. Dilatation of punctum and chronic unilateral conjunctivitis aid the diagnosis. Streptothrix, the usual causative organism, is anaerobic, making cultivation difficult (also, the process is often overrun by bacteria). Direct smear is used for preliminary diagnosis.

2. Streptothrix in direct smear (gram stain). Crush the concretions, add water, smear, flame, and stain. The picture shows gram-positive, unevenly stained, branched filaments. These are segmented into rods and coccoid bodies (spores).

3. *Nocardia*, genus of *Actinomycetaceae*. Grows aerobically and slowly (three to four weeks) on Sabouraud's medium. Colonies are wrinkled, crumbling, and resemble mycobacteria.

4. Nocardia in smear from culture (Giemsa stain). Nocardia fragments readily into bacillary and coccoid elements; some remain filamentous.

5. Leptothrix.

   A. In tissue section (Verhoeff stain). Note slender, granular rods, arranged in clumps.

   B. Smear from film on teeth. Long, unbranched filaments are typical for saprophytic strain.

PLATE XXX 177

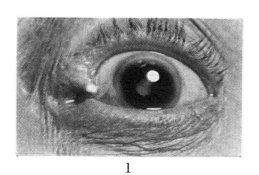

1

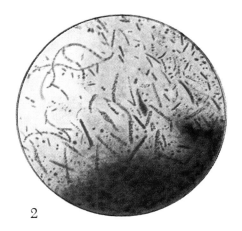

2

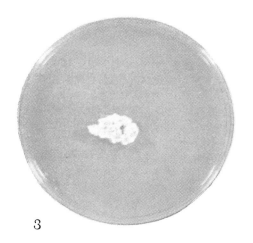

3

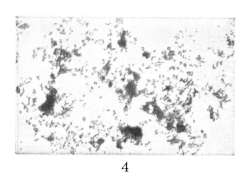

4

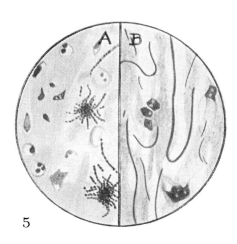

5

PLATE XXXI

1. Mycotic keratitis due to *Candida albicans* (from a case of generalized, fatal candidiasis). Multiple elevated corneal lesions, yellowish and definitely marginated. The process is indolent, with moderate inflammation. Also note multiple, isolated, quiet skin lesions. Diagnosis is confirmed by bacteriologic and experimental studies (see 5, below).

2. Hypopyon keratitis. *C. albicans* isolated. The abscesslike keratitis is ulcerated in the center and covered by a brownish, necrotic mass resembling bread crumbs. *C. albicans* found in corneal scraping (see 4, below).

3. Thrush. Develops after prolonged use of antibiotics. Other lesions on the skin, including the eyelid, are definitely marginated, accompanied by blepharitis and dermatitis.

4. *C. albicans* in original corneal scraping (gram stain) (from patient in 2, above). Yeastlike bodies of *C. albicans* and pseudomycelia are illustrated.

5. *C. albicans* in original corneal scraping (Giemsa stain) (from patient in 1, above). Branching, segmented, beaded pseudomycelia and round or elongated yeastlike cells are found.

PLATE XXXI   179

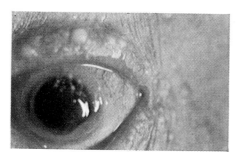

1

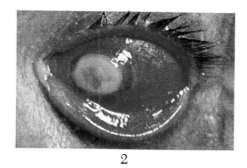

2

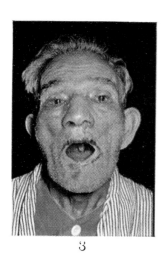

3

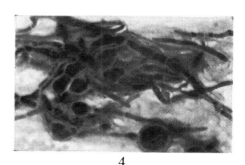

4

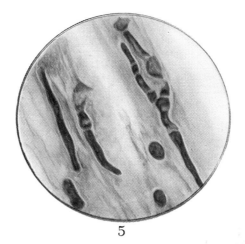

5

PLATE XXXII

1. *Candida albicans* in smear from culture on blood agar (gram stain). Gram-positive, round bodies in cluster arrangement can be distinguished from staphylococci by their larger size, budding, and more intense gram stain.

2. *C. albicans* culture on blood agar. Colonies are small, round, opaque, dry or moist, as are staphylococcal colonies. (Have yeastlike odor and yeastlike morphology.)

3. *C. albicans* culture on Sabouraud's medium. Colonies are cream-colored and soft.

4. Chlamydospores in fresh culture on corn-meal agar (direct examination). Place plate under the low power objective. Examine the peripheral zone of growth covered by a coverglass. Chlamydospores are thick-walled, terminal cells, the resting spores of pseudohyphae. Use corn-meal agar to stimulate growth. Chlamydospores and pseudomycelia indicate a pathogenic strain of *Candida*.

PLATE XXXII 181

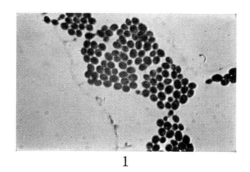

1

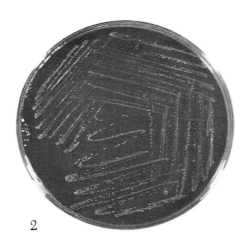

2

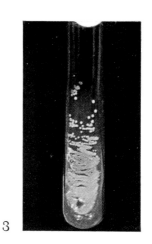

3

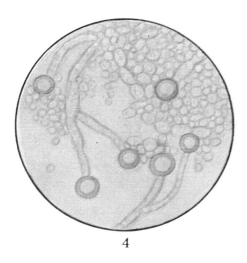

4

PLATE XXXIII

1. Choked disc. Papilledema has occasionally been associated with systemic blastomycosis.

2. *Blastomyces dermatitidis* on Sabouraud's medium. White, cottony colonies later become brownish and prickly, as in center. Growth requires four weeks or more.

3. *Blastomyces dermatitidis* in wet preparation. Budding, double-contoured yeastlike cells typical for this fungus are seen.

4. *Blastomyces dermatitidis* smear from Sabouraud's culture (cotton blue stain). Demonstrates filamentous (mycelial) stage of growth. Long filaments have conidia.

5. *Histoplasma capsulatum* (Giemsa stain). *Histoplasma capsulatum* is shown within mononuclear cell. The oval yeastlike bodies resemble protozoa.

6. *Histoplasma capsulatum* on Sabouraud's medium. Colonies are cottony white, becoming brown in old culture. Growth requires at least three weeks.

7. *Histoplasma capsulatum* subculture on blood agar.

8. *Histoplasma capsulatum* smear from Sabouraud's culture (cotton blue stain). Wet preparation shows typical spherical thick-walled spores with fingerlike projections.

PLATE XXXIII 183

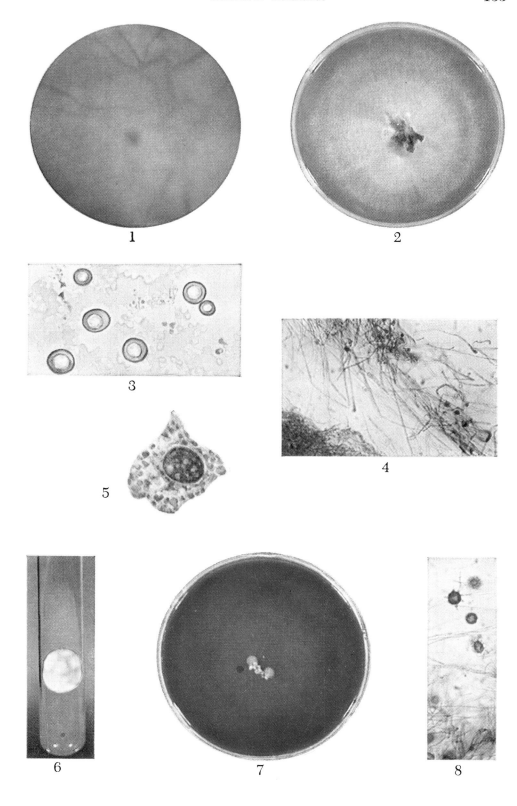

1

2

3

4

5

6

7

8

PLATE XXXIV

1. Granulomatous skin ulcer caused by *Cryptococcus neoformans*. Such local lesions may lead to systemic infection. Cryptococcosis may coexist with other diseases (Hodgkin's disease, sarcoid, etc.), creating a bizarre clinical picture.

2. *C. neoformans* (India ink preparation). This staining method demonstrates the thick walls of the yeastlike cells, important for identification. One cell shows budding.

3. *C. neoformans* on Sabouraud's medium. Colonies are mucoid and slimy, resembling cultures of Friedländer's bacillus.

4. *C. neoformans* culture on blood agar. Gray, opaque, round colonies, resembling staphylococcal colonies. Smear is helpful for differentiation.

5. *C. neoformans* in smear from blood agar culture (Giemsa stain). Polygonal bodies, with honeycomblike arrangement.

6. *C. neoformans* in smear from blood agar culture (gram stain). See description under 5, above.

PLATE XXXIV 185

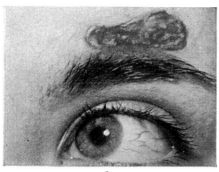

1

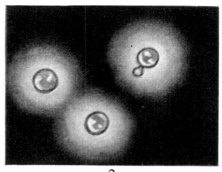

2

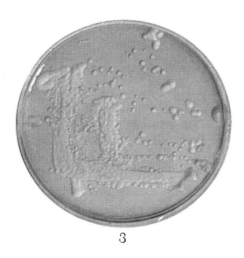

3

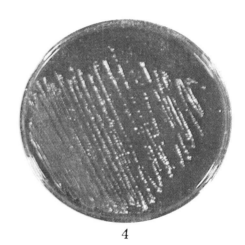

4

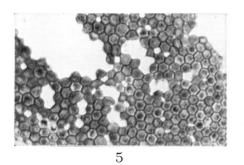

5

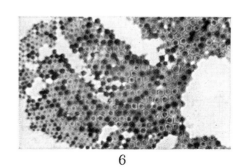

6

5

Miscellaneous Agents

PITYROSPORUM OVALE

Pityrosporum ovale (P.O.) is of particular interest to the ophthalmologist. While it is an almost constant finding in seborrhea, opinions as to its etiologic role are varied. Whether or not *P. ovale* is a cause of seborrhea, its presence is of diagnostic value.

This yeastlike fungus does not produce a mycelium. Because of its lipolytic properties, the organism does not fit into any group.

Morphology. The typical yeastlike budding bodies vary in form, being either spherical, ovoid, cylindrical, or flask-shaped. Round forms may predominate over the oval in the scrapings from the lid margin (Plate XXXV, 2, 3) and in acute process. Flask-shaped forms are more common in dandruff. They are gram-positive and usually stain deeply. Staining with methylene blue is preferable. The slide must be heat-fixed and stained with methylene blue for five minutes. It should be washed carefully during staining, as the greasy specimen may slide off.

The organism is distinguished from staphylococci by its large size, budding forms, and dense gram staining.

Culture. Cultivation of *P. ovale* is extremely difficult because of its lipolytic properties. A great achievement in cultivation was made by Benham. It was shown that wort agar, containing oleic acid, and Littman's agar, with olive oil, are the most suitable media. Growth is more successful on Littman's agar. The colonies have the same characteristics as those of many other yeasts, resembling staphylococci (Plate XXXV, 4). They have a greasy appearance and may float on the oil. A cheesy odor is characteristic. Cultivation is still difficult and often negative. Growth takes about seven days; contaminating molds are not uncommon, and staphylococci or other bacteria are invariably present. Subculture requires about two to five days, and growth can be achieved on Sabouraud's medium (Plate XXXV, 5) or blood agar. Giant colonies may develop.

186

Dandruff or seborrheic scales are used as specimens. As many scales as possible should be scraped from the lid margin, seeded on the plate, then immediately covered with olive oil in a layer 2 to 5 cm thick, sealed, and incubated at 37° C. The growth must be checked frequently.

Seborrhea and P. ovale. Hypersecretion of the sebaceous glands including the meibomian glands is the basis for seborrhea. This lipid secretion is favorable for the growth of *P. ovale*. Although not a cause of seborrhea, the organism may play an important role in its development, either aggravating the process or causing a sensitization of the involved tissue. A number of factors are important in the pathogenesis of seborrhea: systemic disturbances, chiefly of the endocrine system, or constipation, indigestion, excessive use of alcohol or tobacco, some chronic diseases, particularly tuberculosis or syphilis, or familial tendency.

Findings in the Eye. Thygeson was the first to make a thorough study of the relationship of *P. ovale* and seborrheic blepharitis. The evidence concerning its etiologic role was inconclusive. However, he showed a definite relationship between the number of organisms present and the severity of the process.

Seborrheic blepharitis, the basis of which is hypersecretion of the meibomian glands, is the most common type. It is almost always part of a general seborrheic state and is usually associated with dandruff. The condition is characterized by greasy scales (Plate XXXV, 1). Persons of dark complexion have an extensive hypersecretion, and the scales are thick and greasy. The hypersecretion is less in blonds, and the scales are drier.

The condition is often aggravated by secondary bacterial infection, especially *Staphylococcus aureus*. Then the inflammation becomes more severe, the lid margins ulcerate and thicken, and stys and chalazia frequently occur. Seborrheic blepharitis is chronic and may last for years or an entire lifetime. Periodic exacerbations are typical. Hair follicles may atrophy as a result of such a prolonged process, and madarosis may follow. A chronic conjunctivitis usually accompanies the blepharitis. Marginal corneal ulcers are not uncommon.

Treatment. There is no really effective treatment. Local therapy should be combined with general treatment of the seborrheic state, especially the dandruff.

Lid hygiene is of the utmost importance. Cleaning the lid margins with alkaline lotion is suggested before any other local treatment. Twice daily applications of ointment (Thygeson)—1 per cent ammoniated mercury and 1 per cent salicylic acid in petrolatum—may give a good result. Painting of the lid margins with 2 per cent silver nitrate can be used. Expression of secretion from the meibomian glands, followed by massage, is highly recommended. For bacterial infection, suitable antibiotics should be given.

Limiting carbohydrate intake in the diet is also important.

ASPERGILLUS
(*Aspergillus fumigatus*)

Aspergillus is a large genus of fungi widely distributed in the soil, water, air, and animal products. They are the most common and troublesome laboratory contaminants, being frequently found on Sabouraud's medium. Among the many species, *Aspergillus fumigatus* is most often associated with infection, either as a secondary invader or a primary cause of disease. Aspergillosis is frequent in plants, insects, birds, particularly penguins, animals, both wild and domestic, and man. Sometimes it causes great economic loss. The incidence in man is greater in adult males and among workers in an environment contaminated by spores, for instance, squab raisers, furriers using rye flour as a grease remover, or farmers.

Morphology. *Aspergillus fumigatus* may appear in exudate or other specimens as broken fragments of hyphae, together with numerous round, dark green, scattered spores. Culture is needed for identification.

Culture. The fungus is fast-growing at room temperature, with white, filamentous, cottony colonies which become velvety. Later, the colonies are green or dark green, characteristic for spore production.

Diagnosis. Whether aspergillus is a secondary invader or a primary cause of disease is difficult to determine. The presence of spores and their typical arrangements are diagnostically important. They are demonstrated either in wet preparation or in direct examination of the colony. The tube is placed on the stage, and the edge of the colony is studied under the low-power objective. The conidiophore which is characteristic of aspergillus is terminated by a vesicle covered with sterigmata; the latter have long chains of spores.

Pathology. The ear is the most common site of infection. The infection is also found in the orbit and eye, the sinuses, lungs, bronchi, and skin. Aspergillosis is usually a chronic granulomatous process. However, the pathology differs according to the tissue involved. The process in the sinuses and eye is usually pyogenic, resembling bacterial, but distinguished by the periodic appearance of greenish masses containing the fungus. Infection of the nails simulates those of dermatophytes. A mass of the fungus may be found within cavities, a so-called aspergilloma, which can cause obstruction.

Findings in the Eye. Although only a few cases of ocular aspergillosis have been reported, some have been severe, resulting in loss of the globe. Aspergillosis of the orbit, probably a continuation from the sinuses, is known. Fumigatus corneal ulcer, followed by perforation and loss of the globe, has been described by Castroviejo et al. Intraocular post-traumatic aspergillosis has been reported by Rychener. Aspergillosis of the orbit, blepharitis, or dacryocystitis may occur. The incidence of fungal ocular infections is probably much greater than has been diagnosed. Therefore, Birge in reviewing mycotic diseases of the eye, has emphasized that the so-called saprophytic fungi must be re-evaluated.

Treatment. Surgical treatment is usually indicated for localized granuloma, and drainage for abscesses, both followed by iodides. In processes that cannot be treated surgically, slow or rapid iodide therapy is used.

MUCOR
(Phycomycetes)

The mucor fungi, like aspergilli, are constant contaminants in cultures of clinical material. They are widely distributed in soil, manure, and fruits, being commonly known as bread molds. However, the mucor fungus is extremely pathogenic for man, causing mucormycosis in patients with uncontrolled diabetes mellitus. Mucormycosis has been most often described in Germany. It is not transmitted from man to man.

Morphology. The fungus can be readily demonstrated in acid-Schiff, hematoxylin-eosin, and silver preparations, as large, broad, nonseptate, branching hyphae. Because of their thin walls they cannot be stained well by other methods.

Culture. The fungus grows quickly on Sabouraud's medium and fills the test tube or Petri dish with large, grayish mycelia in three to four days. Detailed culture studies are required, since these fungi in cases of mucormycosis have mostly been described post mortem.

Pathology. Mucormycosis is rapidly fatal, within one to five days. The infection is mainly of the brain or lungs. However, the brain can be secondarily involved by initial invasion of the orbit or sinuses. The process is usually characterized by acute inflammation and by vascular thrombi in which the fungus has been revealed.

Findings in the Eye. Acute orbital cellulitis [11] is the most common ocular manifestation of mucormycosis. The process is usually continued from sinusitis and spreads to the brain, causing meningoencephalitis. The associated symptoms are: proptosis, internal hemoplegia, and external hemoplegia. Only three cases of chronic ocular manifestation are known. Two of them are keratomycoses, and one an intraocular mycosis resembling Coats' disease, described by Wadsworth, which was not associated with diabetes.

Treatment. In any suspected case, treatment should be started at once. This includes use of systemic antifungal drugs such as intravenous amphotericin B, oral nystatin (Mycostatin), or potassium iodide. Antibiotics are administered for secondary bacterial infections.

SUPERFICIAL MYCOSES
(Dermatomycosis; Dermatophytosis)

This section is concerned with superficial fungus infections of the skin and its derivatives, such as hair and nails. Systemic involvement is almost unknown. Dermatomycosis is widely distributed, though it has some geographic preference. It is estimated that one half of the population of the United States sooner or later develops this disease.

Fungal species causing the dermatomycoses are divided into three genera: 1, *Trichophyton;* 2, *Epidermophyton;* and 3, *Microsporum.*

Numerous names are confusingly applied either to fungi or to mycoses; their complicated classifications are matters for the mycologist.

The superficial mycoses are rare in ophthalmology. A few comments pertinent to ophthalmology will be given.

Morphology.   This varies in different species. The fungus appears as mycelial fragments or long, branching filaments (from the culture). Mycelia may break up into arthrospores which are spores formed by fragmentation of hyphae; they are arranged in various patterns, such as mosaics, sheaths, or parallel rows, in different species. The study of spores is most important for the individual diagnosis of dermatomycosis.

For microscopic examination, place the infectious material on a slide (with a drop of 10 per cent to 40 per cent potassium hydroxide, depending on species), heat gently to clear material, and examine under a coverglass. Direct microscopic examination is very valuable for the diagnosis. Specific identification can only be done by cultivation.

Cultivation.   Cultivation is on Sabouraud's medium at room temperature, growth taking two to three weeks. The colonies are powdery, cottony, or velvety, and of varying colors—pink, red, white, or brownish.

Pathology.   The fungus infects only superficial keratinized epithelial tissue and grows so superficially that it resembles colony formation on the surface of a medium. The tissue reaction is very mild; light redness, edema, scaling, vesicle formation, and thickening of the keratinized layer may occur. Secondary infection is common. Then the process becomes more severe, resembling pyogenic infection. The regional lymph glands may be enlarged. Tinea is characterized by spread of the fungus circularly from the center; healing from the inside out, it leaves characteristic rings.

Hypersensitivity to fungal products may frequently develop elsewhere on the body, especially the hands, and usually results in the formation of vesicles.

Though dermatomycosis is a superficial process, it may be very troublesome, as it is chronic and often incurable. The fungi are chiefly transmitted from cats or dogs to children. The infections are more severe in tropical countries.

Clinical Features.   The most common type of dermatomycosis is tinea, or ringworm, having ring-shaped lesions. Tinea may occur in various parts of the body. There are distinguished: tinea capitis, tinea barbae or sycosis, and tinea pedis or athlete's foot. The fungus *Microsporum audouini* is commonly found in both man and domestic animals. Any part of the body may be infected. In children, the scalp is especially sensitive, while the feet are resistant; the opposite is true in adults.

Findings in the Eye. Tinea circinata of the lid skin occurs very rarely and is usually secondary to involvement of the face or scalp. Trichophytosis of the lid may show a very slight inflammation which is patchy in appearance; sometimes a purulent ulcer occurs. The mycosis of the lid margin is scaly or purulent, the latter generally caused by a superimposed bacterial infection.

The regional lymph glands may be enlarged. The cilia or the hairs of the eyebrow are often lost as a result of folliculitis of the hair.

Treatment. The infected epithelial structure should be removed and the infected hair epilated. Application of tincture of iodine or ointments, such as salicylic acid, ammoniated mercury, or sodium propionate, has been used effectively. A compress with potassium permanganate solution is recommended.

REFERENCES

1. Andrew, P. F.   Cerebral mucormycosis (phycomycosis): Ocular findings and review of literature, Surv. Ophth., 6:1, 1961.
2. Baker, R. D.   Mucormycosis—a new disease? J.A.M.A., 163:805, 1957.
3. Benham, R. W.   The cultural characteristics of *Pityrosporum ovale:* lipophylic fungus, J. Invest. Dermat., 2:187, 1939.
4. ———   Cultural characteristics of *Pityrosporum ovale:* a lipophylic fungus. Nutrient and growth requirements, Proc. Soc. Exper. Biol. & Med., 46:176, 1941.
5. ———   *Pityrosporum ovale:* a lipophilic fungus. Thiamin and oxaloacetic acid as growth factors, Proc. Soc. Exper. Biol. & Med., 58:199, 1945.
6. Birge, H. L.   The diagnosis of ocular mycotic infections, Arch. Ophth., 46:225, 1951.
7. Castroviejo, R., and Muñoz Urra, F.   Aspergillosis ocular, Arch. oftal. hispano-am., 21:453, 1921.
8. Cogan, D. G.   Endogenous intraocular fungous infection, Arch. Ophth., 42:666, 1949.
9. Donahue, H. C.   Unusual mycotic infection of the lacrimal canaliculi and conjunctiva, Am. J. Ophth., 32:207, 1949.
10. Emmons, C. W.   The isolation and pathogenicity of P.O., Weekly Public Health Reports, 55 (Part 2):1306, 1940.
11. Gass, J. D. M.   Mucormycosis: review, Arch. Ophth., 65:226, 1961.
12. Gots, J. S., Thygeson, P., and Waisman, M.   Observations on *Pityrosporum ovale* in seborrheic blepharitis and conjunctivitis, Am. J. Ophth., 30:1485, 1947.
13. Harley, R. D., and Mishler, J. E.   Endogenous intraocular fungus infections, Tr. Am. Acad. Ophth., 63:264, 1959.
14. Rosenvold, L. K.   Dacryocystitis and blepharitis due to infection by *Aspergillus niger*, Am. J. Ophth., 25:588, 1942.
15. Rychener, R. O.   Intra-ocular mycosis, Tr. Am. Ophth. Soc., 31:477, 1933.
16. Stern, S. G., and Kulvin, M. M.   Aspergillosis of the cornea, Am. J. Ophth., 33:111, 1950.
17. Stratemeier, W. P.   Mucormycosis of the central nervous system, Arch. Neurol. & Psychiat., 63:179, 1950.
18. Thygeson, P.   Etiology and treatment of blepharitis, Arch. Ophth., 36:445, 1946.

19. Veirs, E. R., and Davis, C. T.   Fungus infections of the eye and the orbit, Arch. Ophth., 59:172, 1958.
20. Vidal, F., and Weil, B. A.   Sebaceous blepharosis, Am. J. Ophth., 36:421, 1953.
21. ———— Zeissitis caused by the round Pityrosporum (abstract), Am. J. Ophth., 36:1181, 1953.
22. Wadsworth, J. A. C.   Ocular mucormycosis, Am. J. Ophth., 34:405, 1951.
23. Wright, R. E.   Two cases of granuloma invading the orbit due to an Aspergillus, Brit J. Ophth., 11:545, 1927.

Plates XXXV-XL

Plates XXXVI, XXXVII, and XXXVIII are included to illustrate cases which have no direct correlation with the subject of the book. Some of them, showing allergic conditions, serve for differential diagnosis. Other cases, having unknown etiology, may suggest viral or bacterial origin. A few emphasize the danger of secondary bacterial invasion.

PLATE XXXV

1. Seborrheic blepharitis (sicca). Lashes and brows are heavily powdered with scales—so-called dandruff of lids. Scalp dandruff is always present. *Pityrosporum ovale* is invariably found. The condition is frequently aggravated by staphylococcal infection.

2. *Pityrosporum ovale* (P.O.) in scraping from lid margin (methylene blue stain). Ophthalmic *P. ovale* is predominantly round, while scalp *P. ovale* is flask-shaped. When staining, wash the preparation carefully, as greasy secretion slips off easily. Cultivation is difficult, and scraping suffices for diagnosis.

3. *P. ovale* in smear from culture (Giemsa stain). Spherical forms predominate. *P. ovale* differs from staphylococci in being larger, taking a lighter stain in center, and having budding cells.

4. *P. ovale* culture (Littman's agar plate with olive oil). Seborrheic scales from lid are seeded on plate. Confluented colonies swimming on oil have an oily appearance; otherwise they are similar to many yeasts. Growth takes about seven days.

5. *P. ovale* culture on Sabouraud's medium (with olive oil). Growth is slower than on Littman's agar. Colonies are gray, opaque, and often confluented.

PLATE XXXV   195

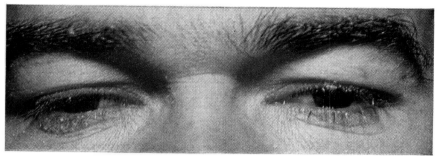

1

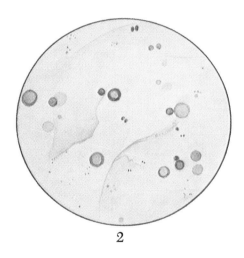

2

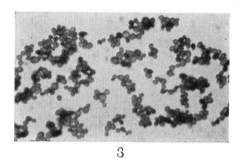

3

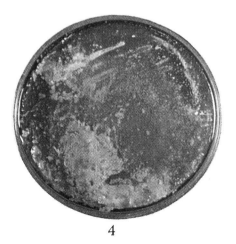

4

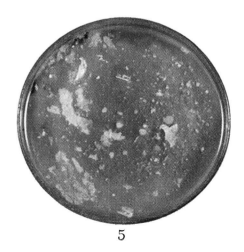

5

PLATE XXXVI

1. *Penicillium* species culture on Sabouraud's medium. Grows readily. Colonies are white, later become bluish green and powdery. Penicillium is a common culture contaminant, occasionally pathogenic. It is rare in eye pathology. It has been recorded as a secondary invader in streptococcal infection of corneal transplant after heavy treatment with antibiotics.

2. Sporebearing hyphae of penicillium. Hyphae, in the form of a brush, have abundant conidia (spores at ends of conidiophores). This structure identifies penicillium.

3. *Aspergillus niger* in culture on Sabouraud's medium. This is the commonest culture contaminant. Occasionally it causes granulomatous infection (sinus, external ear, lung, eye, etc.). In the eye, aspergillosis of the inferior canaliculus, with molasseslike discharge, occurs rarely. Aspergillus may cause granuloma of the orbit (secondary to sinusitis) or hypopyon keratitis (following injury). In both, a molasseslike discharge may be seen. It is difficult to determine the etiologic role of aspergillus.

4. Sporebearing hyphae of aspergillus. Conidia-bearing, unbranched, nonseptate hyphae are needed for identification of aspergillus.

5. Fungi commonly found as laboratory contaminants. Those pictured include aspergillus, penicillium, mucor, and unidentified fungi. Mucor can be an ocular pathogen, usually seen in diabetes. The systemic mycosis is frequently fatal.

PLATE XXXVI 197

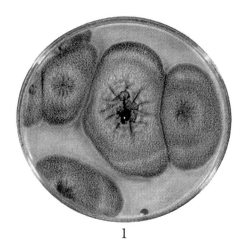

1

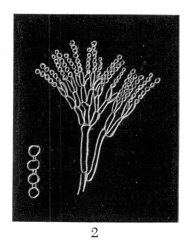

2

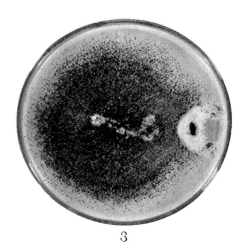

3

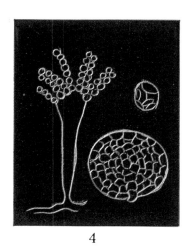

4

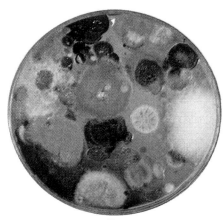

5

PLATE XXXVII

1. Palpebral vernal conjunctivitis (spring catarrh). Marked hypertrophy of papillae, which are hard and flattened. Vascularization of papillae is reticular, resembling petechiae (with slit lamp). Cobblestone and milky appearance differentiates the condition from trachoma. The fornix is not affected. Eosinophils are commonly found.

2. Fibrosis of upper tarsal conjunctiva, consequence of spring catarrh. Results from prolonged process, or overtreatment (particularly with antibiotics) when wrongly diagnosed. Pathologic features: fibrosis, hyaline degeneration, and eosinophilic infiltration.

3. Vernal conjunctivitis, limbal type. Several grayish, limbal lesions of milky appearance, with tendency to confluence. Distinguished from phlyctenules by absence of vascularization and ulceration. Scraping reveals eosinophils. The condition is often associated with Togby's keratitis (epithelialis vernalis), which has a dusty, flourlike appearance.

4. Cytology in scraping from vernal conjunctivitis (Giemsa stain).

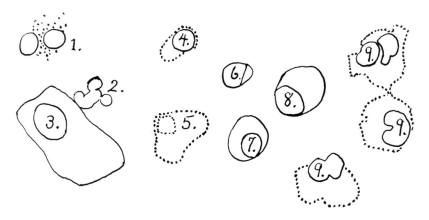

1.		6. Lymphocyte
4.	Eosinophils in various	
5.	stages of development	3. Epithelial cell
9.		
		2. Segmented nucleus of leukocyte, with cytoplasmic autolysis
7.	Plasma cells	
8.		

198

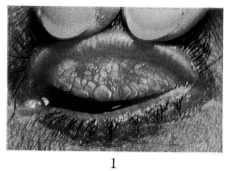

1

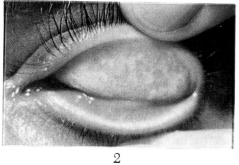

2

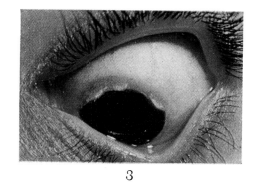

3

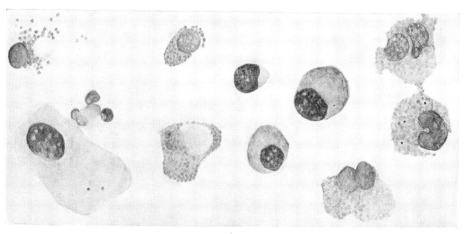

4

PLATE XXXVIII

1. Sclerokeratitis (old healed stage). Keratitis spreads slowly around the limbus, usually associated with scleritis. May be found in tuberculosis or syphilis. Possible allergic origin.

2. Limbal vernal conjunctivitis. Pale pink, quiet lesions show at the exposed area of the limbus (no ulceration, as is usual in phlyctenules). Eosinophils in scraping. Seasonal incidence.

3. Nodular acute unilateral conjunctivitis. Note the distinct round nodules topped by a yellow spot. The bulbar conjunctiva is also involved. Preauricular and submaxillary glands are enlarged. Laboratory tests for bacterial and fungus infections, including leptothrix (in section), were negative. Conjunctival scraping showed eosinophils; the patient's white blood count revealed 10 per cent eosinophilia. An unusual allergic reaction was suggested.

4. Sensitivity reaction to atropine. This may develop after a single instillation.

5. Atopic dermatitis. Shows pustular and exfoliated stage.

6. Cytology in conjunctival scraping (from acute conjunctivitis of toxic or allergic origin).

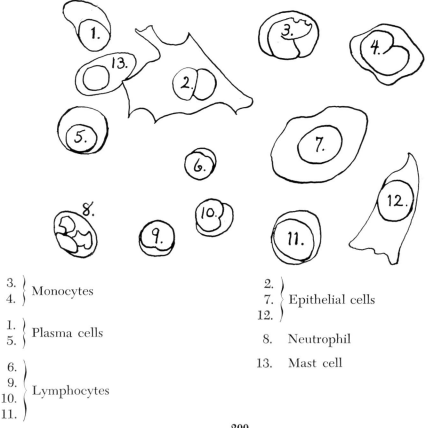

3.
4. } Monocytes

1.
5. } Plasma cells

6.
9.
10.
11. } Lymphocytes

2.
7.
12. } Epithelial cells

8. Neutrophil

13. Mast cell

PLATE XXXVIII

201

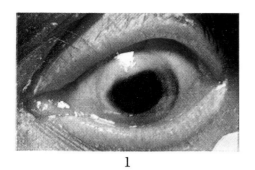

1

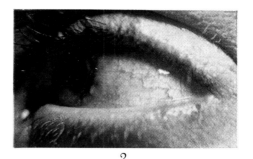

2

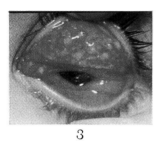

3

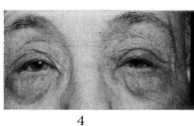

4

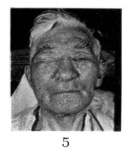

5

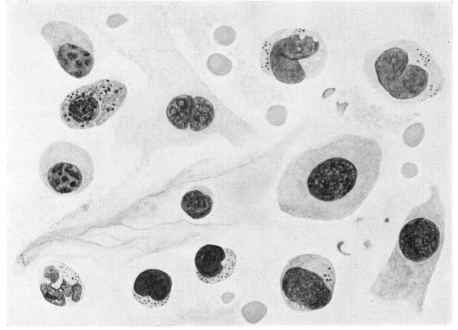

6

PLATE XXXIX

1. Chronic pemphigus of conjunctiva (essential shrinkage of conjunctiva). Beginning of fornix obliteration (usually starts at upper inner angulus). Observe bands of fibrous tissue stretching from palpebral to bulbar conjunctiva. The process is associated with pemphigus of other mucous membranes (rarely it may occur independently). The etiology is disputed. A viral origin is postulated by numerous authors, although without valid proof. Other factors considered are: neurologic, endocrine, and toxic.

2. Hypertrophy of papillae lacrimalis. All four papillae are swollen; puncta lacrimalia are normal. There are a few denuded red spots on neighboring conjunctiva and lid margins. Associated with pemphigus of several mucous membranes; hence it is suggested as an extremely rare pemphigus manifestation.

3. Chronic pemphigus of conjunctiva (associated with pemphigus of other mucous membranes). Following rupture of bullae, the conjunctiva shows a few denuded areas. The epithelium is not repaired; it becomes replaced by fibrous tissue. Note a few large retention cysts, possibly resulting from duct blockage by shrinkage. Unlike bullae, the cysts are thick-walled and persist. Bullae are extremely thin-walled, appearing and disappearing quickly.

4. Chronic ocular pemphigus in late stage. Extensive formation of scar tissue, followed by almost complete obliteration of lower fornix (total symblepharon). Note keratitis at lower limbus, due to exposure. Primary keratitis in pemphigus is rare.

PLATE XXXIX 203

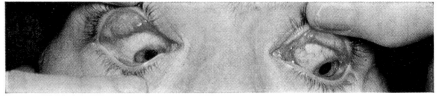

1

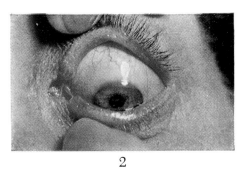

2

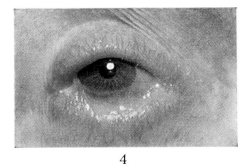

3

4

PLATE XL

1. Anterior staphyloma (bulging iridocorneal scar). The bulging scar is the consequence of an expanded perforated ulcer (iris is the main constituent). Picture demonstrates a thin scar with underlying pigment showing through.

2. Folliculosis (adenitis of conjunctiva: Duke-Elder). Abundant, large, discrete, semitransparent, pinkish yellow follicles. They are arranged in rows, mainly in the lower fornix, and are not found on bulbar conjunctiva. Lack of inflammation and absence of trachomatous inclusion bodies are important for differentiation. It is mainly a disease of childhood. The condition may exist undetected for months or years, especially in institutions.

3. Marginal degeneration of cornea. A vascularized furrow, usually bilateral, running along the limbus and separated from it by a narrow clear zone. It may be superimposed on arcus senilis. A frequent sequela of this condition is ectasia or perforation. (Note ectasia as dark area on upper part of furrow.) Bacterial complication is particularly dangerous.

4. Leproma of cornea. General appearance of patient with corneal leproma (described in Plate XII, 5).

5. Rodent ulcer (Mooren's ulcer). A chronic, superficial corneal ulcer, of unknown etiology, occurring in the elderly. Laboratory diagnostic tests are negative. Simultaneously with the ulcer's advance, the peripheral portion of the lesion heals, with heavy vascularization.

6. Lye burn. A catastrophic occurrence in which liquefying necrosis (unlike coagulative necrosis from acid) develops rapidly, often within a few minutes. This case showed abundant white discharge, with complete destruction of the conjunctiva and cornea. Even in apparently mild burns, destruction may later develop; cautious prognosis is advised. Laboratory diagnosis is mandatory, to rule out bacterial infection.

7. Leukoma of the cornea, sequela of bacterial keratitis. Dark spot shows cystoid degeneration (usually resulting in fistula).

8. Cystic distention of lacrimal sac, sequela of chronic dacryocystitis.

PLATE XL 205

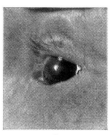

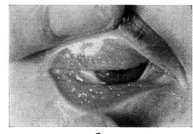

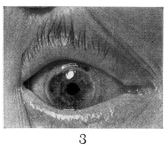

1

2

3

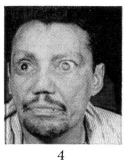

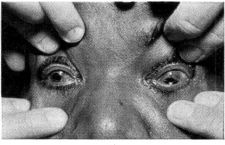

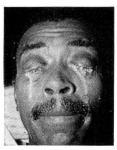

4

5

6

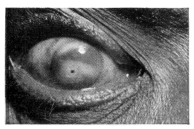

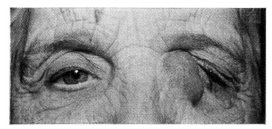

7

8

6

Technic of Laboratory Procedures

SMEAR

Smears are used primarily for the study of bacteria and exudates.

Obtaining Conjunctival Smear (Plate XLI, 1). The discharge should be taken from the conjunctival surface only. This avoids contamination from the angulus or lid margins where saprophytic staphylococci and *C. xerosis* are almost constant inhabitants. If necessary, these areas can be investigated separately.

Flame a loop and let it cool. Pass this sterilized loop over the lower conjunctival fornix two or three times in the same direction. To remove excess fluid, tap the loop a few times on the slide, away from the center. This is quicker than waiting for the excess to evaporate. The exudate, which is the important material, usually sticks to the loop. It appears as a small, flocculent mass which should be smeared on the center of the slide. To get a proper gram stain, it is absolutely necessary to smear the material diffusely and evenly. In uneven smears gram-negative bacteria may appear as gram-positive or the reverse. If the material is sticky and thick, a loopful of sterile saline should be added.

To fix the material, pass the back of the slide over the flame three or four times. Avoid overheating, which can destroy bacteria and cells.

Obtaining Smears from the Lid Margin. The technic varies with the condition. 1, Squamous blepharitis (scraping is preferable, but swab can be used): rub a dry swab over the lid margin. Place the specimen, if it is dry, in a drop of saline on the slide, then smear. (A wet swab also can be used.) 2, Ulcerative blepharitis: using a wet swab, remove all scales and crusts from the edges of the lids. Then use a dry or wet swab to obtain the specimen from the base of the ulcer. Smear as in 1. 3, Angular blepharitis: the material should be smeared from the external angulus and prepared as in 1.

Obtaining Meibomian Secretions. The general principle involved is to express material from the meibomian glands. Place a suitable firm support, such as an applicator, behind the lid margin and press. Special expressers are available for this purpose.

Obtaining Lacrimal Canaliculus Specimen (Plate XLI, 6). This technic is particularly important when one is considering the diagnosis of fungus infection. The conjunctiva is anesthetized, and a support is put behind the canaliculus which is then pressed. In this way, a specimen may be expressed. If large concretions are encountered, the canaliculus may have to be split. Once obtained, the concretions are to be crushed, saline added, and the smear prepared. Fix the smear by flaming and stain the specimen with the gram or Giemsa stain.

Obtaining Lacrimal Sac Specimens (Plate XLI, 7). It is important to express material from the lacrimal sac in the proper fashion. Doing this should be routine for every ophthalmologist. The secretions of the sac can be obtained by firm pressure over the sac. While applying pressure, one must observe the lacrimal punctum, which has first been everted and cleansed. In this way, even a scanty secretion will not be missed if it should roll into the fornix. It should be stressed that in hypopyon keratitis examination of the lacrimal sac contents must not be overlooked.

Obtaining Smears from Corneal Ulcers. Topically anesthetize the cornea. Remove all exudate and necrotic material from the ulcer crater. (The causative bacteria are usually found under the necrotic material.) This is best done with a moist swab. The specimen is then obtained with a dry swab or, if one prefers, a loop. In deep ulcers be particularly gentle so as to avoid perforation. In serpiginous ulcers (usually pneumococcal) the specimen is obtained by looping material from beneath the undermined progressive margin. Smear the obtained material, flame it gently, and stain by gram or other technic. This technic is used to obtain material both for the smear and for the culture.

SCRAPING

The technic of scraping is important for several reasons: it permits detailed studies of the cells, inclusion bodies, and cell response to various ocular diseases, especially viral or allergic. It is also an important tool in the diagnosis of bacteria having an intracellular habitat. Scraping is most valuable in the active phase of the disease, before secondary changes take place.

Technic. Topical anesthesia is applied to the eye; 0.5 per cent Pontocaine is the anesthetic we use. Many others are of equal value. The anesthetic drops are given two times or even more, depending upon the patient's response and the disease process. A thickened or scarred conjunctiva may require more drug than a conjunctiva of more normal dimension.

It is obvious that the preferred site for scraping is the area involved in the disease process, for example the upper tarsal conjunctiva in trachoma or the lower tarsal conjunctiva in inclusion conjunctivitis.

The instrument we use is a specially made platinum scraper approximately 0.5 cm wide. The scarificator or other instrument can be used.

Scraping the Conjunctiva (Plate XLIII, 1, 2). Take scrapings from the tarsal conjunctiva of both lids, near the retrotarsal conjunctiva and about 2 mm away from the lid margin. The latter is a transitional area characterized by naturally keratinized epithelium which may mistakenly be considered as pathology. The technic is the same for both lids, except have the patient look down to evert the upper lid, and look up to evert the lower.

First, swab off excess discharge; then scrape, passing the spatula two or three times in the same direction (not back and forth). Do this thoroughly but avoid bleeding. The handle of the spatula should be inclined in the direction of the stroke or held perpendicularly to the conjunctiva. To avoid corneal injury, do not allow any part of the spatula blade to be free in front of the cornea. Remove excess fluid from specimen by tapping spatula on the edge of the slide. Place spatula flat; pass back and forth until cohesive material appears, then spread evenly and gently (Plate XLIII, 3, 4). Never use flaming, which destroys the fine structure of the cells, but fix immediately in absolute alcohol. Various kinds of alcohol are used for fixation, but it must be absolute. In our laboratory absolute methyl alcohol has been constantly used, with complete success. Let the slides stand in a staining glass filled with absolute alcohol (capacity 70 cc) for five minutes; remove and allow to dry, then stain with Giemsa stain (Plate XLIII, 5).

A description of staining technics can be seen on page 218.

Corneal Scraping. Care must be taken to avoid injury, but material should always be obtained from the tissue actually infiltrated. Use only the angular part of the scraper, as shown in Plate XLI, 5. For site of scraping, see directions for corneal smear, above. Prepare two slides, one for gram and one for Giemsa or other stain.

Obtaining Scraping from Lid Margin (Plate XLI, 3, 4). This is needed chiefly in seborrheic blepharitis. The patient must close both eyes. Pull lid sideways and hold; this makes the lid margin less movable. Then scrape scales from roots of lashes, along the lid margin. Spread scales on the slide, adding a drop of water if the preparation is too dry. Flame, and stain with methylene blue (five minutes) or with the gram stain. Wash slide carefully during staining, as the greasy specimen may wash off. In ulcerative blepharitis, first remove crusts, cleanse off excessive exudate, scrape, smear, and stain with gram stain.

The drugs used to anesthetize before scraping may dilute or wash off a scanty exudate and, in some infections, can interfere with the growth. Therefore, the smear and culture are best obtained before the use of drugs.

Plates XLI-XLIII

PLATE XLI

1. Obtaining conjunctival specimen (loop technic). Pass the loop across the lower conjunctiva two or three times in the same direction (not back and forth). The gram stain requires a smooth, even specimen on the slide.

2. Obtaining conjunctival specimen (swab technic). Use a dry or wet swab to obtain culture specimen. If the discharge is abundant, this technic is useful for the smear as well. Absorb material (do not rub).

3 and 4. Scraping lid margins. Pull the lid sideways and hold. Scrape from the roots of the lashes along the lid margin. (In ulcerative blepharitis, first remove the crusts.) Spread this material on the slide, adding water if the material is dry. Fix and stain by the gram stain or by Neisser's stain (see pages 218, 220).

5. Corneal scraping. Anesthetize the cornea. Use only the angular part of the scraper (carefully, to avoid injury). If the border of the ulcer is undermined, use a loop to get into the pocket. In an abscesslike ulcer, clean out the necrotic material and scrape the base. Prepare slides for gram and Giemsa stains.

6. Lacrimal canaliculus specimen technic (usually necessary in fungus infection). To obtain a specimen, place a suitable support behind the canaliculus and squeeze. Crush the concretions, add saline, and smear. Flame; stain by the gram and Giemsa methods (see pages 218, 219).

7. Obtaining specimens from lacrimal sac. Clean the inner angulus and evert the punctum lacrimalis (or scanty secretion may be missed). Then press the lacrimal sac.

8. Reagents for gram staining. Left to right: 2 per cent solution of gentian violet, iodine solution gram, 95 per cent alcohol, 1 per cent solution of safranin. (Keep bottles always in the same order.)

PLATE XLI

211

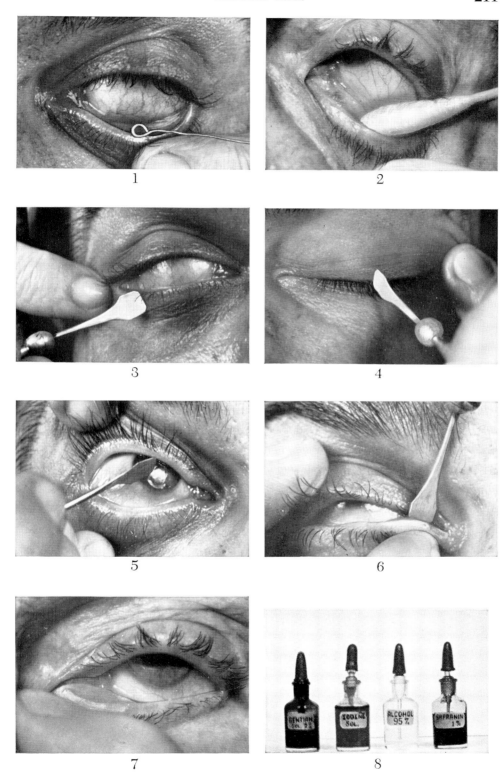

PLATE XLII

1. Tray with simple equipment for preparation of specimens.

One wide-mouthed, screw-cap jar for sterile swabs.

Two dressing jars: one for slides in 95 per cent ethyl alcohol (for scrapings), the other for dry slides (for smears).

One dressing jar for sterile droppers (dropper discarded after one use).

Bottle containing sterile anesthetic.

Bottle containing normal saline.

Wide-mouthed glass container for scraper, loop, glass pencil, forceps, and red wax pencil.

2. Inoculation of specimen on blood agar (or any plate of solid medium). Streak on plate by rolling the swab (away from edge, as peripheral part could be air-contaminated).

3. Disk sensitivity test (Difco Bacto Unidisk, Code 7002, is used here). Place Unidisk on plain or blood agar inoculated with the culture.

4. Mannitol fermentation. Positive fermentation (yellow) differentiates pathogenic staphylococci from saprophytic staphylococci.

5. Inoculation on Sabouraud's agar (for fungus isolation). Flame the mouth of the tube; spread specimen from bottom almost to top. Fungi usually grow best at room temperature. (Avoid dryness and too much light.)

6. Inoculation of Brewer's thioglycollate medium (supports both facultative and strict anaerobes). The photograph illustrates an error often made. The correct way is to break off the applicator below the cotton plug (hold over flame). A large inoculum is needed. Rotate gently to mix the culture.

7. Glucose-maltose-sucrose test. Basic carbohydrate tests used in laboratories, particularly for *Neisseria* and *Corynebacterium* genera. In the case illustrated, the organism tested is glucose-positive (yellow), maltose and sucrose-negative, typical for the gonococcus.

8. Candle jar. For description, see Plate XVIII, 5.

PLATE XLII

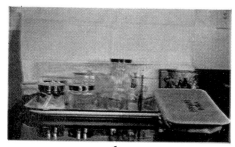

1

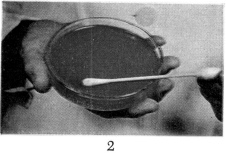

2

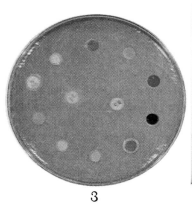

3

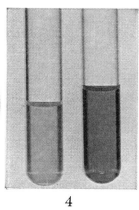

4

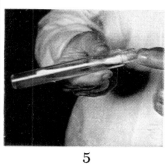

5

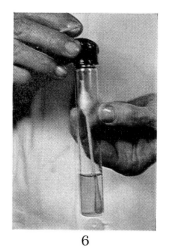

6

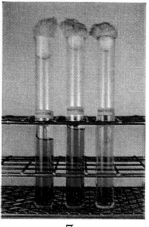

7

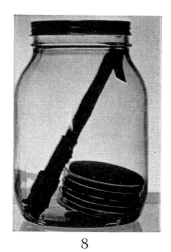

8

PLATE XLIII

1. Scraping of lower conjunctiva. Anesthetize the conjunctiva. Flame a spatula and let it cool. Have the patient look up. Pull the lid down with a finger placed at the cilial margin. Swab off the exudate, then scrape, passing the spatula two or three times in the same direction (not back and forth) firmly, but avoid bleeding. Spread the specimen evenly on the slide. Fix in absolute methyl alcohol and stain by the Giemsa method (see page 219).

2. Scraping of upper tarsal conjunctiva about 2 mm behind lid margin. (Here, keratinized epithelium is normally present.) Have patient look down. Pass spatula in a direction away from the lid margin; be careful to avoid the cornea.

3. Technic for spreading the scraping. Remove excess fluid from the specimen by tapping the spatula on the edge of the slide. Place the spatula flat; pass it back and forth until cohesive material appears; spread this evenly and gently. Mark the patient's initials on the slide with a glass pencil.

4. Density of scraping.

5. Giemsa staining (Thygeson's modification). Fix the slide in absolute methyl alcohol for five minutes. Stain in a Coplin jar by diluted Giemsa stain (1 drop Giemsa solution to 2 ml distilled water). Place in an incubator for one hour; without an incubator, the process requires two or three hours. Dip each slide first in one jar of 95 per cent ethyl alcohol, then in another. Allow the slides to dry, and examine them under the oil immersion objective (see page 219).

6. Microscope with oil immersion objective in place for use.

PLATE XLIII 215

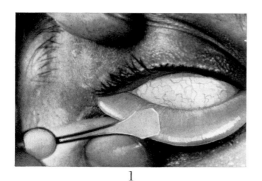

1

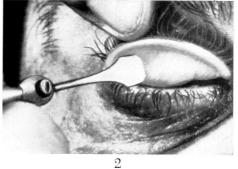

2

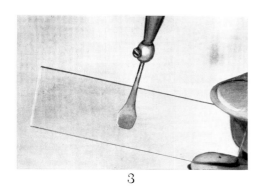

3

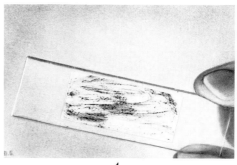

4

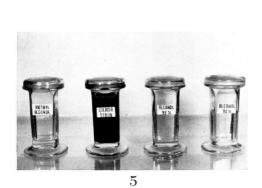

5

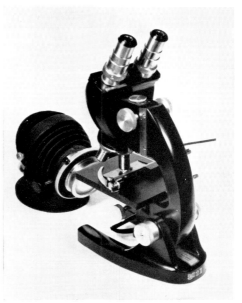

6

CULTIVATION

Though a great variety of media exist, it is impossible for the average laboratory to deal with more than a few. Anyone doing ocular bacteriology needs to become proficient in handling a certain number of media. Recent work indicates that we must be on the lookout not only for bacteria but for fungi as well, and therefore we must also be able to handle fungal media.

Blood agar is the basic medium used in ophthalmology. Most ocular bacteria will grow on this medium. However, if clinical manifestations so indicate, media such as Brewer's medium (thioglycollate) (Plate XLII, 6), which can be used for both aerobic and anaerobic bacteria, or chocolate agar, Löffler's serum, and carbohydrate media (Plate XLII, 7) must be utilized. A preliminary smear of the discharge may aid one's choice of a particular medium. Cultivation of fungi is described in that section (page 159).

If the identification of microorganisms requires a complicated procedure, the specimen had best be sent to a general bacteriology laboratory.

CULTURE

Even if the process is not bilateral, specimens from both eyes must be cultured. In the unilateral process, a comparison with the normal eye is necessary, or the normal flora of the inflamed eye could, by mistake, be considered the pathogen. For reasons of economy, in our laboratory we divide each plate into four sections, thereby using it for cultures from both eyes of two patients. If proteus is suspected in the diagnosis, use a plate for one patient only, or the entire plate will be overgrown by this organism.

The lower fornix is the usual site for obtaining the specimen. Use a wet or dry swab to absorb material, touching the conjunctiva three or four times as you roll the swab along the fornix. Do not rub, and avoid contamination from the lid margin and lashes. It should be emphasized that a wet swab often becomes contaminated, requiring frequent control and sterilization. Therefore, use a dry swab if the material is to be cultured immediately.

To streak on the blood plate, twirl the swab gently, taking care not to dig into the medium. Start away from the edge (Plate XLII, 2), as the peripheral part could be air-contaminated; in such cases, tiny colonies of the contaminating organism may not be noticed. Place in the incubator for 24 hours at 36.8° C to 37° C., not higher. If the culture is negative or scanty, reincubate for another 24 hours. This is especially necessary if pneumococci, streptococci, the Koch-Weeks bacillus, or the neisseria group is suggested. Use a candle jar if indicated. Subculture is often necessary for identification.

Use the medium indicated, as is given in the description of species. A specimen in the amount of a full loop must be streaked on a suitable solid medium or dipped into a suitable fluid medium.

In mixed culture, separation of microorganisms is always difficult. Of the many methods, the simplest is Koch's plating method. For this, a little material and dry plates are necessary. Two streaks about 10 mm apart are crossed at right angles (one each way). It is often advisable to do this over a second or even a third plate without recharging the loop.

Identification of Colony. The colonies are best examined during the first 48 hours of incubation. Later, they may become degenerated and not be typical. In describing colonies, attention should be paid to shape, size, and other factors. Changes in the medium, such as hemolysis and liquefaction, should be evaluated. Other factors to which attention should be paid are structure, color, transparency, surface, consistency, and emulsifiability. The odor is significant for some species.

Bacterial motility to a great extent determines the characteristics of the growth. Some motile bacteria, such as proteus, swarm in a continuous film on a solid medium. Other motile bacteria move in a clockwise or counterclockwise direction, being closely packed.

As a rule, study of a colony merely indicates the group to which the organisms belong; it does not usually differentiate the various species of the group. For the latter, see descriptions of the species.

A few general characteristics may help to roughly differentiate the colonies of gram-negative organisms from gram-positive. Colonies of gram-negative bacteria (on blood agar) are usually not very opaque, are more confluent and more mucoid than gram-positive colonies, and generally develop an odor.

Smear from the Culture. A smear of the culture may help to identify the microorganism. Several different colonies can be examined on the same slide. First, mark a few circles on the slide with a glass pencil. A wax pencil is not recommended, as during staining its granules wash out onto the slide and may be confusing. To prepare a homogeneous suspension, place a drop of water beside each circle, then lightly touch the loop containing the bacterial specimen in the center of the circle. Flame the loop to remove excess. With the same loop, add a little water to the material in the circle and emulsify. Then spread evenly and thinly. With a small colony that is not well isolated, fishing under the low-power objective of the microscope is necessary.

Fix the slide by flaming, and stain with the gram stain or other indicated stain.

STAINING REACTION

The staining reaction of bacteria, particularly their response to certain differential stains might be regarded rather as a chemical test than a demonstration of structure. Usually, the entire cell is uniformly stained; in some

bacillary forms, the ends of the bacteria may be more deeply stained
(polar stain). Some bacteria, such as corynebacteria, stain unevenly (due
to metachromatic granules), resulting in barred or beaded forms. Irregular
staining is also characteristic of acid-fast organisms.

As a rule, to identify organisms by morphology and staining reaction is
impossible. However, presumptive diagnosis in association with the clinical
picture is feasible. For instance, in tuberculosis, acid-fast organisms can be
identified as tubercle bacilli. The gram-negative kidney-shaped cocci of
ophthalmia neonatorum are usually gonococci. Stout diplobacilli in scrapings from a corneal abscess are easily identified as a *Moraxella* species.

Routine stains are gram for bacteria; Giemsa for cell structure; methylene blue for *Pityrosporum ovale* or neisseria; acid-fast for *M. leprae, M.
tuberculosis,* and some fungi; cotton blue stain for certain other fungi.

Numerous other stains are used for special purposes, for instance, to
demonstrate capsules, flagellae, or metachromatic granules.

GRAM STAIN

1. Gentian violet (2 per cent water solution), for 1½ minutes. Cover
entire smeared specimen without excess, but sufficiently.

2. Wash with water.

3. Apply iodine solution gram for 1½ minutes. Pour off solution. Do not
wash with water.

4. Decolorize in 95 per cent alcohol. Put on alcohol, shake slide, and
pour off very quickly. Do this two or three times, until gentian stops washing off.

5. Wash with water immediately after above.

6. Stain with safranin (1 per cent water solution for 1½ minutes or
more).

7. Wash with water.

8. Blot, dry, and examine under oil.

There are many modifications of the gram method. For practical
reasons, we simplify the staining procedures. The gentian violet water solution is used, and we time each staining procedure uniformly for 1½ minutes.
For good results, the decolorization has to be very carefully done and, most
important, the specimen spread thinly and uniformly on the slide.

Gram staining is of great value to distinguish two groups, gram-positive
and gram-negative organisms. The method, however, is not always accurate.
Gram-negative organisms frequently retain the stain and may appear to be
gram-positive, as the gonococcus. The reverse is true with gram-positive
organisms; they may fail to retain stain in old culture. Dead or degenerated
cells alter completely their physical and chemical properties.

GIEMSA STAIN

1. Fix air-dried slide in chemically pure acetone-free absolute methyl alcohol for 5 minutes.

2. Dilute (in special staining jar) Giemsa stain (best is Hartman-Leddon Company's). Use 1 drop of stain to 2 ml ordinary distilled water for injection. This has been used satisfactorily even without testing of reaction. Put slide in jar and place the staining jar in the incubator for *1 hour*.

3. Decolorize in two changes of 95 per cent ethyl alcohol for 5 seconds each. Dry in air and examine under oil.

For successful staining of thin films, alcohol must be absolute (methyl or other), water of neutral reaction, and fixation not less than 5 minutes.

Giemsa stain is used primarily for the study of cytology in scrapings. It is important for diagnosis of allergy, inclusion bodies, and cell response. We found also that the structure of some fungi, particularly filamentous, can be better revealed.

If rapid diagnosis is required, especially in allergic conditions, the Wright stain is preferable.

METHYLENE BLUE STAIN

1. Fix the slide by passing it through the flame three or four times.
2. Stain with methylene blue for 5 minutes.
3. Wash with water.
4. Dry, and examine under oil.

The stain is especially suitable for *Pityrosporum ovale* in seborrheic blepharitis. The greasy specimen is easily washed off, and a gentle procedure is required.

ACID-FAST STAIN (ZIEHL-NEELSEN)

1. Fix the slide by passing it through the flame three or four times.
2. Apply Ziehl's carbolfuchsin solution.
3. Gently steam the slide by careful heating for 3 to 5 minutes with intermittent replacement of the evaporating carbolfuchsin solution.
4. Wash with water.
5. Decolorize with acid alcohol until only a slight suggestion of pink remains.
6. Wash with water.
7. Counterstain with Löffler's methylene blue for ½ minute.
8. Wash with water.
9. Dry and examine under oil.

CAPSULE STAIN (HISS METHOD)

MATERIALS:

1. *Gentian violet or fuchsin solution*
   Saturated alcoholic solution of gentian violet or
   basic fuchsin .   .   .   .   5 ml
   Distilled water .   .   .   .   95 ml
2. *Copper sulfate solution*
   Copper sulfate .   .   .   .   20 gm
   Water .   .   .   .   100 ml

The best source of material for the demonstration of capsules by this method is infected exudate from the animal body. If a stock culture is to be examined, the organisms should be emulsified in a drop of serum on the slide.

TECHNIC:

1. The film is dried but not fixed with heat.
2. Flood the glass slide with gentian violet or fuchsin solution.
3. Hold the preparation for a second over a free flame until it steams.
4. Wash off the dye with the copper sulfate solution. (Do *not* wash with water.)
5. Blot.

LACTOPHENOL COTTON BLUE MOUNTING MEDIUM

This stain is used (in moist preparation) for most fungi. It can be purchased ready-made.

1. Put a drop of this medium on the slide.
2. Add specimen of fungus. Tease fungus with dissecting needle.
3. Examine under a coverslip.

NEISSER'S STAIN

1. *Methylene blue (Neisser's)*
   Methylene blue .   .   .   .   1 gm
   Alcohol, 96 per cent .   .   .   .   .   .   20 ml
   Glacial acetic acid .   .   .   .   .   .   50 ml
   Water .   .   .   .   950 ml
2. *Bismarck brown*
   Bismarck brown .   .   .   .   1 gm
   Water .   .   .   .   100 ml

For staining Klebs-Löffler bacilli and *C. xerosis* to show metachromatic granules. Use a 24 hour culture on blood serum. Make films and stain with methylene blue for one-half minute. Wash in tap water and treat with Bismarck brown for one-half minute. Wash, dry, and mount. The metachromatic granules stain very dark; the bodies light yellow.

Index

221